# PROFESSIONAL HYPNOTISM MANUAL

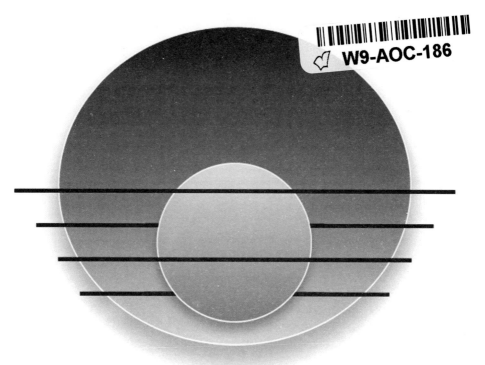

*Introducing Emotional and Physical Suggestibility and Sexuality*

by John G. Kappas, Ph.D.
California Licensed Marriage and Family Therapist
Founder, Hypnosis Motivation Institute

7th Edition 2015

7th EDITION 2015 PUBLISHED BY:

**PANORAMA PUBLISHING COMPANY**
18607 Ventura Boulevard, Suite 310
Tarzana, California 91356 USA
800-634-5620

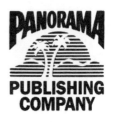

Library of Congress Card Number: 78-107043

Printed in the United States of America

# DEDICATION

I dedicate this manual to my associate and friend, Christina Vick, for her dedicated persistence in pushing me to write and helping me to compile this material.

# ACKNOWLEDGMENT

The staff and students of the **HYPNOSIS MOTIVATION INSTITUTE** asked the hard and searching questions that compelled me to expand and refine these theories. Then, when they were satisfied, they took what I offered and fully and completely applied it to their personal lives, as well as in colleges, hospitals, and clinics nationwide.

I gratefully acknowledge their tremendous help and support.

# TABLE OF CONTENTS

## CHAPTER 10 – SELF-HYPNOSIS

# FOREWORD

Dr. John Kappas' *Professional Hypnotism Manual* is more than just another book about hypnosis. It is, instead, a comprehensive system for examining human behavior under the umbrella of "subconscious behaviorism." In this text, Dr. Kappas completely redefines our understanding of hypnosis and how it works with his "message-unit theory of hypnosis" and his revolutionary model of "Emotional and Physical Suggestibility and Sexuality." The "E&P" model provides hypnotherapists with a roadmap for tailoring hypnotic suggestions to match the individuality of the client's communication style and personality type. These new concepts, along with the countless gems of practical wisdom contained in this book, have earned the book distinction as a classic text of modern hypnosis.

Dr. John G. Kappas (1925-2002) unknowingly distinguished himself as the Father of the Hypnotherapy profession in America when, with the help of the AFL/CIO International Union, he authored the definitions of "Hypnotist" and "Hypnotherapist" for the Federal Dictionary of Occupational Titles. The introduction of these titles into the Federal Dictionary in 1973 marked the official recognition of the professional practice of hypnosis and the title of "Hypnotherapist" in the United States.

Dr. Kappas' influence on the profession of hypnotherapy in the United States expanded further in 1987, when the nonprofit organization, the Hypnosis Motivation Institute (HMI), founded by Dr. Kappas in 1968, achieved distinction as the first hypnotherapy college in America to become nationally accredited by an accrediting agency authorized by the U.S. Department of Education. In 2006, HMI's accredited college began offering, free to the public, an online streaming video course titled "Foundations in Hypnotherapy," based on the teachings in this text and featuring vintage footage of Dr. John Kappas.

The continued popularity of this streaming video course, along with the *Professional Hypnotism Manual*, clearly demonstrates that Dr. Kappas' material is as useful and valid today as it was when originally published in 1975. HMI's college and clinical internship continues to rely on Kappas' *Professional Hypnotism Manual* as the foundation for its accredited training courses. Throughout his 32-year career, Dr. Kappas maintained an unwavering focus on, both, his private-practice clients and the constant refinement of his concepts through teaching in the HMI classroom. The Ivory Tower academician would be well-advised to consider the practical implications of Kappas' approach to therapy and his empowerment of the masses to become helping professionals.

George J. Kappas, M.A., M.F.T.
Director, HMI College of Hypnotherapy

# CHAPTER 1 – A CONTEMPORARY APPROACH TO HYPNOSIS

## INTRODUCTION

It is not my intention to bore the reader with the ancient history of hypnosis because I believe that the real story of hypnosis is here and now. What has been recorded up to this point has always been reiteration from one writer to another. Much of it has been based on fiction, doubt, superstition, and negativity, and has nothing to do with what the person interested in the modern uses of hypnosis really wants or needs to know.

Hypnosis, as we know it today, began in the 1950s, and will probably not come into total acceptance until the 1980s. When the history of hypnosis as a successful therapeutic medium is recorded, it will address the innovative idea of *suggestibility*, a behavior all humans possess. It will be referred to as *hypnotic suggestibility* – *hypnotic* referring to a receptive state, and suggestibility referring to how a person learns. Hypnotic suggestibility will be defined as *receptive learning* and will become increasingly recognized and used as a major tool in all the healing arts and in educational institutions. The history of hypnosis will show how receptive learning is now used, and how it will continue to be used in many facets of our lives, in almost all areas of teaching, in positive-thinking groups, religion, metaphysics, meditation, and advertising. The history will also describe the associations, the unions, the professionals, and the lay individuals who have contributed so much to hypnosis and have used it to educate and bring help and understanding to millions.

There are two people from the early history of hypnosis who deserve mention because they initiated major trends. The others, including Freud, simply followed their lead. Franz Anton Mesmer, the man who gave hypnosis its original name, produced his first theories of Mesmerism in 1765. He believed that he possessed the power to magnetize people into his control, and during the 1780s, he acquired many followers. Some accepted the concept of magnetism, while others believed that the state of control characteristic of Mesmerism resulted from other factors, noteworthy among them the personality of Mesmer himself.

One who disbelieved the theory of magnetism was Dr. James Braid, a physician of the 1840s, who believed that Mesmerism was a suggestible state resembling a nervous sleep. Today, Mesmerism bears the title that Braid gave it – *Hypnotism* – from a Greek word meaning *sleep*. While observing hypnotized subjects, Braid found that many physiological changes took place. The most obvious change, of course, was the rapid-eye movement characteristic of the light stages; then the change in breathing and the subsequent passivity as the subject entered a deeper state resembling sleep. He noticed that during this state, the subject was easily influenced by verbal suggestions, even to the point of controlling many of his involuntary functions. Braid tested his subjects by giving them suggestions in the waking state as well as in the hypnotic state, and he concluded that the subjects appeared to be more receptive in the hypnotic state.

Since then, we have recognized that many different suggestible states exist and that subjects respond differently in each of them. We have further determined that these various states can be created by understanding the difference in suggestibility from one subject to the next.

## WHAT IS HYPNOSIS?

In order to understand what creates the hypnotic state, we must first understand primitive man, his development, and his means of survival.

As animals evolved, the survival instinct caused them to develop an increased ability for either *fight* or *flight*. Some developed greater strength and aggressiveness (fight), while others developed agility, speed, and increased sensitivity of the senses of smell, sight, and hearing (flight). Animals that did not develop the ability for either fight or flight, but remained passive, have become extinct. During his early evolutionary stages, man survived and functioned totally on instinct. He did not have the inhibitory processes of guilt, shame, embarrassment, sense of morality, religious conditioning, faithfulness, and obligation. He defecated and urinated without thought wherever he happened to be, screamed or expressed aggression when he was threatened, had sex anywhere or with anyone, whenever the urge was present, and ran or fought according to the size or sound of his enemy. When he could not run or fight, he would retreat into a passive, apathetic state and play dead until the threat was over.

Because of his small stature and because of the natural weapons of his animal enemies, he had to develop the ability to use objects available to him, such as sticks and stones; and he made clothing from skins, which served as natural camouflage. In order to avoid detection when he was hiding, he had to limit his defecating and urinating habits to certain areas within safe compounds where he lived and was beginning to group. Thus, he began to develop the first inhibitory processes: covering nakedness, confining defecation and urination, and grouping into units for protection.

The evolution of these inhibitory mechanisms progressively brought about greater consciousness, and with greater consciousness came more responsibility to others, as well as to himself. His subconscious responses then started to handle everything that was involuntary, which came to include the inhibitory mechanisms. The inhibitory processes further developed into an automatic compensating system called the *parasympathetic nervous system*. Whenever the preparation for fight or flight took place through the *sympathetic nervous system*, the parasympathetic system would regulate the sympathetic back to normal. As man evolved and fight became less socially acceptable, the parasympathetic system began to suppress the fight reaction, allowing flight to become the more acceptable escape mechanism.

At this point, he began to form anxieties because he was developing a consciousness and could not escape back into primitive mind. Therefore, whenever he faced message units that were consciously unknown or were known to be threatening, he attempted to regress back to primitive behavior, rather than use the new conscious area of mind. This escape mechanism has remained constant to the present time, although it has become more difficult to escape as consciousness has expanded. The reason for this is that, by pure habit of coping with the continually increasing societal pressures, man has developed a stronger resistance to flight.

Hypnosis and anxieties are brought about in the same way. It is our experience that many people who are in a high-anxiety state will escape the anxiety by entering into a trance state – a reversion to a more primitive area of mind.

The human being receives messages into his brain through four sources. The first, the external environment, sends message units dealing with such things as the weather, the news, music, television shows, jobs, interaction with partners, and anything else from our everyday surroundings that affect us. The second source is our body. Its normal tensions, movements, digestive activities, feelings of tightness, pains or discomforts, all constantly send message units to the brain. The third source is the conscious mind, which handles our logic, reason, objectivity, decision-making, and all of the influencing factors that affect us consciously. The fourth, and probably the most influential source, is the subconscious mind, which receives and holds, without accepting or rejecting, all the message units we receive from our religious, social, and genetic backgrounds and all the little conflicts that enter our consciousness daily.

Through his evolutionary development, man has acquired the ability to deal with these message units without triggering the primitive fight or flight mechanism. He has been able to accomplish this by adding tolerance to the fight or flight reaction, thereby extending it to deal with the Pain/Pleasure Syndrome that a more modern society imposed on him. This modern syndrome deals with knowns (pleasure) and unknowns (pain). A known is a unit of communication that does not represent any threat because it has been learned or experienced before; we can associate with it, understand it, and be comfortable with it. An unknown is just the opposite. Because it has not been learned before, it causes us to experience psychological and physiological reactions that we are not used to. These reactions threaten the brain and body, and the resulting fear brings us pain.

What is known to some may be unknown to others; so what is pain to some may be pleasure to others, and vice versa. Even physical discomforts or negative feelings, such as depression, can be classified as pleasurable for some people, simply because they have been experienced before and the mind will accept them as knowns. This is why the mind will accept negatives.

In order to cope with the increasing number of message units coming at him from all four areas (and based on the Pain/Pleasure Principle), modern man extended his tolerance to the fight reaction by adding *Reaction vs. Action*, and to the flight reaction by adding *Repression vs. Depression*. Had he not evolved in this manner, he would have had only one way out when the message units became too great to handle – to escape by denying reality. He could not do this, however, for the denial of reality would not provide him with acceptance and would consequently deprive him of pleasure and bring him pain. This pain would come from lack of social acceptance. The desire for social acceptance, then, motivates the individual to cope with, and adapt to, reality.

As society presents more and more challenges that the involuntary system cannot handle well, some reactions cease to be involuntary and, instead, come into the conscious control. As man expands his consciousness, his involuntary system depends less and less on itself and more and more on the consciousness to feed back information for reactions. So, the more complex society becomes and the more threats it poses, the greater the conscious control, and the fewer the subconscious reactions. As more knowns accumulate during this expansion of the consciousness, the tolerance of pressures increases.

With the extended fight syndrome of *Reaction vs. Action*, the human developed nervous anxiety and tension. A reaction would take place in the body and the individual would attempt to vent it out by walking, running, working, or taking some physical action. The extension of the flight syndrome involved *repression* (taking everything inside, hoping to vent it later through dreams or emotional reactions) or *depression* (an escape into fantasy or deep, long sleep). The modern extension of these reactions does not, however, eliminate the possibility of triggering the primitive modes of fight or flight. We may revert back to these primitive reactions whenever the message units are too great to be handled by the modern syndromes or whenever we experience a feeling of loss of control.

For instance, should certain circumstances take place where one or more of the four sources send too many message units, we will become threatened and begin to feel insecure in our external environment. If we find we cannot cope with the pressures of the times or of the moment, more message units than normal begin to move into the brain. Then the body begins to tighten and malfunction. When we cannot keep up with external message units, our body begins spasmodic shivering, and the adrenal glands start to secrete. As the body develops more pressure, more message units also move into the brain, and this reflects into the conscious mind, which will now try to develop more logic and reason to work it out. When the conscious mind can no longer handle the input of message units entering the brain, the subconscious immediately prepares us for fight or flight. The heart pumps faster, blood pressure goes up, blood is forced from the organs to the muscles, and the pupils dilate. But when we realize that there is nothing to fight, this physical feeling increases the anxiety and creates apprehension and fear of the unknown, causing a pressure buildup inside. In its effort to protect us, the self-regulatory parasympathetic nervous system then overcompensates, by changing this fight or flight physical reaction to a slow, passive condition, where we lose the will to fight and remain still and sleep-like in a depressed, apathetic state until the danger passes. This reminds us of the time when threatened primitive man and animal would lie very still and play dead until the predator left.

In other words, when we find out that we cannot fight the environment, we cannot fight the job, and we cannot fight the messages that are coming into our brain, we revert back into the escape mechanism of flight, which immediately puts us into an apathetic, depressed, hypersuggestible state. This can create futility and melancholy, if it happens in an uncontrolled situation because the inhibitory processes become totally disorganized and we become overly receptive to negative input. As a result, we overreact to all our senses and have a loss of tolerance.

Hypnosis is created by the same mechanism, but in a positive controlled situation. For example, a subject who has never been hypnotized enters the unfamiliar external environment of an office where hypnosis takes place. The expectation is building and the environment of the hypnotic surroundings is sending added message units into his brain. He is beginning to develop some fears of the unknown, and may experience nervousness, feelings of loss of control, or fear of exposure. He is led to sit in a comfortable chair and is instructed to close his eyes, removing the sense of sight (one of his protective devices). The operator begins to feed message units into his brain by telling him that his arms, legs, and entire body have a tendency to feel heavier and more relaxed. More message units bombard his body. He may find that his body is beginning to relax – a change from what he felt a few moments ago – and more message units move into his body. Should an arm-rigidity or an arm-raising be induced, more message units will be put into his brain from his body. The conscious mind immediately tries to fight this condition, but finds that it cannot because the operator is usually speaking faster than the subject's conscious mind can digest the information without confusion. In addition, the operator is using misdirections, capitalizing on the subject's expectations, emotional feelings, and ego sensations, and using phrases that are new to the subject.

The subject now reverts to his subconscious mind and the defense mechanism of fight. He may find himself abreacting and may find his body tightening, when he realizes that, during this particular state, a certain part of his brain is already inhibited. The many incoming message units cause him to seek out the escape mechanism of flight; and at the sudden moment of truth, when the subject is jarred slightly by a snap of the fingers, a touch on the forehead, or just an increase in the operator's tone of voice, the escape takes place, replacing the urge to fight, and immediately inducing a hypnotic state in the subject. The message units going into the brain create the anxiety that eventually leads to the escape process, which is hypnosis. At this time, the body and brain feel safe within their environment, and the brain loses the critical ability that might otherwise cause it to reject suggestions.

During this fight or flight reaction in hypnosis, we see obvious physiological changes taking place. The first is the change of breathing, as the brain requires more oxygen to help in dealing with a new and fearful situation. The second change is dryness in the mouth area, also common in fear reactions. The third, and most obvious, is the rapid eye movement, as the brain tries to fight by simulating dream venting. Once the subject enters the hypnotic state, the body becomes still, the eyes have a tendency to roll upward, the breathing slows down, and the facial muscles relax, just as they do when an anxiety reaches a peak and the escape mechanism of depression takes over. This lethargic, limp, state is apparently triggered by the release of a relaxant chemical, the same as the one that is triggered by the suggestion of relaxation.

In summary, anxiety and hypnosis are the same, except for one characteristic: hypnosis is a pleasurable state within a controlled environment, whereas anxiety is a worried, fearful state within an uncontrolled environment. When over-activity of the senses takes place, causing extreme receptiveness, the hypnotized subject is guided with positives, while the anxious person is guided by his own negativity.

## THEORY OF MIND

There are four areas of the mind that must be affected before a person can enter a hypersuggestible state:

**1. THE CONSCIOUS MIND** – Retains and remembers the events and feelings of approximately the past one-and-a-half hours only.

**2. CRITICAL AREA OF MIND** – Part is conscious; part is subconscious. Contains memories of approximately the past twenty-four hours only. Any time a suggestion is given to a subject that is detrimental to his well-being or in total opposition to his way of thinking, he will critically reject it by abreacting.

**3. MODERN MEMORY AREA OF MIND** – Part of the subconscious mind. Holds memory from conception to present in this life.

**4. PRIMITIVE AREA OF MIND** – Part of the subconscious mind. Includes all the primitive memory that lies dormant, including genetic heritage and evolved learning and conditioning. Will react only when triggered, regressed, or threatened beyond the point of reason. Examples would be a fight or flight reaction or an impulse to kill. Suggestions affecting this area result in rapid reaction without reason.

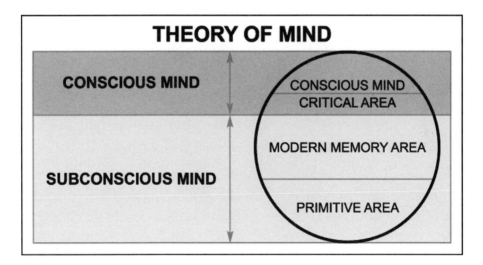

The message units from a normal day's input enter the conscious mind first, and then pass into the conscious portion of the critical area. Here they accumulate and are held. Critical area is partially conscious and partially subconscious because we have been educated and conditioned to develop an analytical sense of evaluation on the conscious level. At the same time, we have learned on a subconscious level to avoid anything that is critical or threatening to us. The critical area will not analyze message units or release them into the modern memory area, as long as consciousness is present, but only when sleep takes place or the consciousness is in abeyance, as in the hypnotic state because, at that time, there is no conscious critical ability to hold onto them.

If too many message units accumulate in critical area, the body fatigues and starts preparing the person to go into a sleep state to vent. The brain may become disorganized, making the individual fatigued, irritable, and upset. The more emotional traumas any individual has, the more sleep he needs. Considerable trauma gives rise to the so-called *depressive sleep*.

Once a person goes to sleep, accumulated message units are immediately dropped into the subconscious mind. Here they are critically analyzed and some are allowed to go into modern memory; others are discarded (vented) through dreams. Those that lie in modern memory, eventually begin to filter into different areas of primitive mode.

If the person receives an overabundance of message units when it is impossible to sleep or escape, hypersuggestibility and the accompanying anxiety result. At this time, the critical area becomes less critical (because it is being threatened and because the consciousness is simulating sleep in this hypersuggestible state) and starts dropping message units without evaluating them. This creates negative habits and increases hypersuggestibility.

The average person stays awake at least sixteen hours, so the conscious mind has roughly sixteen hours to evaluate message units, before they are allowed to go into the modern memory area. The longer it takes a suggestion to reach the modern memory area, the weaker it becomes. The strength and longevity of any suggestion depends on how quickly and how often it is received in the modern memory area. The longer it stays in the critical area, the more it becomes distorted and weakened. This means that it takes a long time to consciously create a suggestive pattern from the day's input.

In hypnosis, this whole process takes place in minutes. From the conscious mind, a suggestion moves into the critical area, where it is critically analyzed. Because there are so many unknowns going into the subject's mind, the critical mind usually quickly drops the suggestion into the modern memory area. In some instances, the subconscious mind may attempt to abreact a suggestion and vent it out through the body. However, if that suggestion is repeated after the abreaction is recognized and there is no following abreaction, the suggestion goes to the modern memory area. Once a suggestion is accepted in the modern memory area, it returns to the critical area and then to the conscious mind for final acceptance and acting upon.

When the conscious mind is unconscious, as in sleep, it is not receiving anything. It is only dropping the message units into the subconscious and venting them through dreams. In hypnosis, the conscious mind is not unconscious, so it is able to receive, as well as drop and vent message units. The release of message units into the subconscious mind takes place instantly, as the consciousness goes into abeyance, and then the venting process through hypnotic suggestions begins.

A suggestion given in the hypnotic state is much stronger than one given in the conscious state because it moves so quickly from the critical area to the modern memory that it does not have time to become diluted. Further, if a consistent positive reaction to a suggestion takes place, that reaction will become a permanent habit, and constant willpower and motivation will not be necessary to maintain it. The success of the suggestion is predicated on how it is understood going from the conscious mind to the critical area (where it is critically analyzed and possibly changed) to the modern memory area (where it is accepted as a symbol) to the final stage (where it is acted upon). Success is also dependent upon how well the structure was prepared prior to giving the suggestion. Structuring or building a foundation means giving the subject known reasons as to why a suggestion will take hold, achieving proper *desensitization* if a conflict (fear or negative learned habit) exists, and giving literal or inferred suggestions according to the subject's suggestibility.

*This page intentionally left blank.*

# CHAPTER 2 – CHARACTERISTICS OF EMOTIONAL AND PHYSICAL SUGGESTIBILITY

## THEORY OF EMOTIONAL AND PHYSICAL SUGGESTIBILITY

Hidden deep in the mind of every hypnotist is a nagging question that comes up every time a subject does not respond as the hypnotist expects or desires. This question has been rationalized, analyzed, and lied about, but still remains. "Why do some subjects respond to hypnotic suggestions and depth, while others do not?" The answer was discovered a decade ago.

For many generations, hypnotists have divided suggestibility into three different stages: Hypnoidal (light), *cataleptic* (medium), and *somnambulistic* (deep). They believed that the deeper the subject, the better the results the hypnotist could obtain. A cataleptic subject would achieve better results than a hypnoidal subject, and a somnambulistic subject would do best of all. The 60% or 70% of the population that fell into the category of suggestibility that they believed to be lighter than hypnoidal was dismissed as being unhypnotizable.

Since 1967, when the Hypnosis Motivation Institute recognized the existence of two distinct types of suggestibility – *Emotional* and *Physical* – a new hypnotic world has been revealed. Human behavior has led us to recognize that *everyone* is suggestible to something; some to physical sensations, others to emotional stimuli, still others to environmental stimuli, and some to all three. This new information has opened doors to the hypnotherapist, the motivator, the counselor and to anyone using hypnosis for self-improvement.

To explain Emotional and Physical suggestibility, we will begin with a diagram:

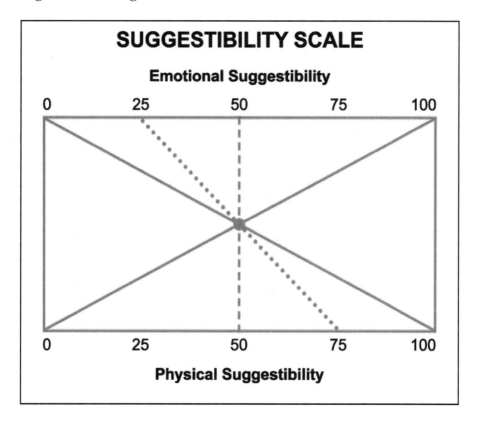

The line with its upper end at 100 and lower end at 0 represents the 100% *physically suggestible* subject. He will respond to any direct, literal suggestion affecting his body, but will not respond to suggestions affecting his emotional behavior.

The line with its upper end at 0 and its lower end at 100 represents the 100% *emotionally suggestible* subject. He will respond to all suggestions affecting his emotional behavior, but will not respond to suggestions affecting his physical body or physical movements. This type of subject does not respond well to direct, literal suggestions, but is very responsive to inferred suggestions and misdirection.

A line drawn between the two 50s (dotted line on diagram) represents the *50/50* subject (50% Emotional and 50% Physical).

This type of subject has traditionally been called a *somnambulist*. He is the best subject for stage hypnosis because he responds to physical challenges, emotional suggestions, positive and negative hallucinations, amnesia, anesthesia, and time distortion. There are relatively few people with this type of suggestibility. Although it can be developed over a period of time, it is not necessary for good results in hypnotherapy.

Not all subjects fall into the extreme Emotional or Physical categories. There are subjects with every possible combination of Emotional and Physical suggestibility, from 1% Emotional and 99% Physical to vice versa. To see a diagrammatic representation of any combination, locate the known score (either Physical or Emotional) on the Suggestibility Scale, connect that point with the point where the triangles touch, and extend the resulting line to reach the line of opposite suggestibility. The individual's full suggestibility is now graphically demonstrated. For example, the starred line on the Suggestibility Scale represents a 75% Physical/25% Emotional subject.

In addition to Emotional and Physical suggestibility, there is a sub-category of Emotional suggestibility called *intellectual suggestibility*, which is present in only about 5% of the population. The Intellectually suggestible person is one who must have a reason for everything. If you tell him that when you hypnotize him, he will feel calm and relaxed, he will ask you why. When you give him suggestions in hypnosis, he will ask why they will work. You can usually reach him only through inferred suggestions, and must always give him a reason for the suggestion and a reason why it will work. The *auto-dual method* of hypnosis is the most successful with a subject of this type. If you tell him to repeat everything after you and assure him that he is really conducting the session himself, he will usually respond more readily than if you intellectualize every statement you make to him.

In the past, only Physical suggestibility was recognized. Consequently, it was believed that the depths attained in hypnosis by a Physically suggestible subject were the only true indications of the hypnotic state and that the methods used to hypnotize a subject were the same for everyone. In addition, 60% to 70% of the population was considered unhypnotizable. We now know that these unresponsive subjects were Emotionally suggestible and that hypnoidal, cataleptic, and somnambulistic stages of hypnosis for Emotionally suggestible subjects are quite different than for those who are Physically suggestible. The *emotional somnambulist* (100% emotional) responds with the same intensity to suggestions affecting his emotional behavior as the physical somnambulist (100% Physical) responds to suggestions relating to his physical body, but his reactions are not as immediately obvious. The Emotional somnambulist appears to be in a very light state of hypnosis, or not to be in the hypnotic state at all, while the Physical somnambulist exhibits all the characteristics formerly attributed to the somnambulistic state. In fact, *natural somnambulists* (50% Physical and 50% Emotional) were not even distinguished from Physical somnambulists in the past because both have the same appearance in the hypnotic state. The difference between them, however, is vast because the natural somnambulist will respond equally to suggestions affecting his emotions and his physical body, and not just to one of the extremes.

The understanding of Emotional suggestibility has expanded the scope of hypnosis, by taking it out of the guessing stage and allowing us to work with a great many people with whom we could not previously work. Emotional suggestibility was discovered through accident, determination, and ego. In trying to prove to ourselves that an individual could be hypnotized, we discovered how to develop and use inferred inductions with methods of misdirection that were effective with certain types of subjects who were not responding to the usual methods.

A question often asked by hypnotists is: "Why does a subject enter hypnosis very quickly and deeply one day and only very lightly the next?" We now know that the answer is that on one day the operator happened to use inferred suggestions for the entire induction, and the next day he used literal suggestions. He probably achieved success with inferred suggestions by accident because he, at least partially, recognized that the subject was not responding well to his customary literal suggestions. When he finally began to correlate which suggestions were affecting which subjects and why, successes became more frequent and more enduring.

Once we recognized Emotional suggestibility and learned how to hypnotize this type of subject, we found that he is far more receptive to therapy than the Physical subject, who responds well to physical tests and, on the surface, appears to be the better subject. The reason for this is that therapy usually does not deal with physical problems. In most cases, it deals with emotional problems or with physical problems that have been created by emotional problems, in which case, the emotional problem is the cause and the physical manifestation becomes the symptom. In therapy, you must create Emotional suggestibility, if it is not already present, in order to affect emotional problems the client may be having. Unfortunately, most modern-day hypnotists are totally unaware of the existence of Emotional suggestibility, and are, therefore, unable to help the people who are the most receptive to hypnotherapy.

In essence, suggestibility is a person's hypnotic personality, determined by all of the conditioning and all of the experiences he has had throughout his life, particularly the experiences of the first six to eight years of life. A person becomes suggestible to one extreme or the other because of a defense against either the emotional or the physical. He develops this defense to protect himself from rejection by either his physical or his emotional side, whichever is more vulnerable.

The suggestible pattern of an Emotional is based on a defense to protect his physical body. He will put his emotions out first, before he will accept physical touch. In other words, when he is faced with uncomfortable physical contact, attention, or pain, or if he senses he is about to be put in such a position, he responds with emotions of embarrassment, fear, anger, apprehension, emotional irritation or frustration, as a line of defense to protect his physical body from discomfort. He is especially susceptible to this threat because he tends to be overly concerned with what others think about him, and his embarrassment level relating to his physical body is easily reached. Only if the threat turns out to be unfounded or nonexistent and he finds that he can accept positive emotional feelings, will the defense mechanism lessen and his capacity for physical acceptance increase. The end result of the Emotional's defense is that he develops a habit of suppressing feelings in the physical body, and his ability to feel ego sensations diminishes. The extent of this suppression, of course, is relative to his degree of Emotional suggestibility.

The Physical, unlike the Emotional, uses his physical body as a defense to protect his emotions. He will respond to physical touch with pleasure and has a great need for it, as it represents acceptance to him. He expresses himself bluntly and is not overly concerned with how others see him. When he becomes involved with explaining something, he tends to be animated in movement and gestures and to move close to the person to whom he's talking. He will usually dominate a conversation, barely listening to what the other person has to say. He may cut someone off in the middle of a sentence, in order to get a point across. Whether he recognizes it or not, he has difficulty understanding the emotions of others because he can relate only to what he feels and not to what others say and feel. Because he relates to physical communication, he attempts to reach others through physical closeness and body language and suppresses his ability to relate verbally on more than a surface conversational level. Only when he has achieved enough physical acceptance to ease his urgency and make him feel comfortable, can he open up to positive emotional communication.

The Physical speaks inferentially and understands literally; the Emotional speaks literally and understands inferentially. Even though the Emotional wants to sit back and listen and prefers not to put himself in an embarrassing situation or fight for a chance to speak, and even though the Physical prefers to carry the conversation, a communication barrier will arise between the two opposites. The Emotional will begin to feel frustrated because his suggestibility will not allow him to speak with ease until he is comfortable emotionally, and the Physical's contact needs prevent the Emotional from being at ease. The Emotional will also feel that the Physical is not truly understanding him. In such a situation, the Emotional will tend to close off and withdraw into himself. When deprived of closeness and contact, the Physical will become even more aggressive in order to obtain the physical acceptance he needs to protect himself against emotional rejection. This breakdown of communication, due to differences in suggestibility, is the basis of many friendship, family, and relationship problems.

A clear-cut distinction between Emotional and Physical suggestibility will be difficult to achieve if you confuse – as many do – the way a Physical or Emotional responds with the way he would *like* to respond. Both feel the loss of not being able to experience the opposite of their suggestibility, and they do search for the missing opposite. It is not what a person wants that indicates his suggestibility, but what he has been conditioned to consider threatening, pleasurable, or painful. Every Emotional is potentially capable of feeling everything physical, and every Physical is capable of emotional communication, but they have simply not learned how.

An understanding of suggestibility is imperative for every hypnotist because it allows him to select appropriate inductions for each individual. Emotional inductions and Physical inductions will produce the same beneficial results, as long as each is carefully matched to the individual client's suggestibility and needs.

## HOW SUGGESTIBILITY IS LEARNED

Any given interpersonal message is composed of three parts: the verbal content, the extraverbal (or nonverbal) content, and the state of mind of the receiver. The verbal part refers to the words and their dictionary definition only. For example, consider the common remark, "Isn't it a lovely day?" Without knowing the extraverbal content of this message, we must take it at face value and assume that it is, indeed, a lovely day. The extraverbal part of the message is the sum total of the speaker's gestures, expressions, and bodily attitudes that accompany the verbal message. If the verbal message above was given while the speaker was slumped in a chair with his head in his hands, we would assume that it was an awful day and that the disappointed speaker was being sarcastic when he called it "lovely." If the speaker of the same message was smiling, bouncy, and glowing with excitement, we would assume that it is, indeed, a glorious day. The receiver of any interpersonal message must then interpret both, the verbal and the nonverbal parts of the message, based on how he feels at that particular moment. If he is happy and positive, he is more prone toward an affirmative interpretation; if he is depressed, he is likely to take the negative meaning, even if the extraverbal language does not confirm it.

A person's adult suggestibility, or the way he receives and interprets input, is predicated on how he was communicated with from infancy to adulthood. Of particular importance are the years up to the age of eight.

From the time they are born, until they are two or three years of age, all children are basically Physically suggestible – they reach out for, and touch, everything, in order to gratify their physical and mental curiosity. By the age of two or three, a child will have learned verbal communication, and he will learn about his world through the words instead of through physical grasping. From this time onward, the child's primary caretaker (usually his mother) is responsible for setting his pattern of suggestibility. The child becomes closely attached emotionally and physically to the image of his mother and tries to become like her. As he matures, he will have the same type of suggestibility that she does, although it may vary in degree. If the child's mother uses words of affection (verbal content), treats him affectionately (nonverbal content), and does not suppress his free verbal expressions, the child learns something valuable: what mother says is what mother means, and what she says is a reliable indicator of how she feels about him at the time she spoke. This produces Physical suggestibility. Once begun, this Physical suggestibility becomes exaggerated if the mother remains consistent in saying what she means and following through on her promises. By so doing, she is eliminating any threats to the child's basic physical needs. Her ability to communicate literally indicates that she is Physically suggestible and, as indicated earlier, the child's suggestibility will be similar to hers.

The disciplinary patterns of the mother also greatly influence and reinforce the suggestibility patterns of the child. If, for instance, she scolds and spanks the child when he has done something wrong, but then follows the spanking by holding, caressing and consoling the child, he will come to view the affection and physical touch as compensation for the unpleasantness of the punishment. Eventually, he will develop a habit of searching for this compensation, hoping to eliminate the scolding completely. He learns to dissociate himself from the scolding; and this tendency carries over into adult life, where he continues this characteristic of tuning out when he does not want to hear something unpleasant. Because physical touch is emotionally pleasurable for the child, he becomes motivated to reach for it. That which is uncomfortable for him (scolding and spanking) is ignored, in order to concentrate on what is comfortable. The absence of pain is pleasure, and although pleasure might be only a minimal feeling, it is accepted as pleasurable because of the absence of pain. A Physical is constantly searching for rewards. When discipline is followed with the rewards of touching, the child soon learns that he will be rewarded for doing something wrong. Consequently, he may disobey when he wants affection. The spanking may even become a form of reward because it is associated in his mind with physical touch, a pleasurable feeling to him.

Physical suggestibility is also reinforced if the mother starts off giving physical attention to the child (hugging, kissing, touching) and then changes and rejects him physically. Or, if she overly protects or embarrasses him in front of his friends by constantly cautioning him to be careful ("Wear a coat, or you'll catch a cold"; or "Don't run, or you'll fall."), she could cause him to be overly suggestible in relation to his physical body. Military schools and the military service also reinforce Physical suggestibility.

There are many things that can cause a child to become Emotionally suggestible, but, usually, it is a combination of factors. If a child is in a situation where the mother (or whoever was responsible for communication learning) is ambiguous or contradictory, or where her expression is threatening or negative, the child's understanding will become distorted, and he will develop a defense, whereby he will begin to suppress communication. If his mother makes statements that she subsequently contradicts by her actions (as in breaking a promise), or if the verbal and nonverbal parts of her speech do not express the same thing (as in saying, "Sure, I love you" with clenched teeth), the child will begin to search for the real message under the verbal layer. His suggestibility is then predicated on inference, and he will be affected by what he thinks his mother *really* means by statements or words. Additionally, he will have doubts about how she really feels about him.

Another common cause of Emotional suggestibility is a mother who is overly possessive, and who overwhelms her child to the point where he feels he has to avoid being handled physically. Also, if he is spanked often for things he does not feel he is guilty of and is afterwards ignored, or if he is ignored totally, eventually touch becomes like a spanking. If you reach out to touch him, it causes the same reactions as if you reach out to spank him. He develops a negative association with touch, and protects himself against the unpleasantness of touch (now associated with spanking or with physical smothering), by reacting with defensive emotions, such as, fear and anger, in any situation where he anticipates touching. He does not have a reward associated with touch, as the Physical does, so the absence of touch becomes the closest to a reward he receives. He seeks simply to avoid the pain or unpleasantness, but never receives the gratification that a Physical seeks and receives from touch. Instead, he escapes into what he is most comfortable with – the defensive emotions. The anticipation of a spanking after every scolding causes him to put up an emotional defense to avoid the physical discomforts that will follow. In extreme cases, he may even reach the point where he will block the pain and not even feel the spanking. If he continues to suppress his feelings, he closes off the physical body; and as he grows up, he becomes Emotionally suggestible.

Balanced suggestibility (equal amounts of Emotional and Physical) can result from one of two things: moderate discipline by the mother, coupled with an assurance of love and security, or discipline so inconsistent, that the child develops a basic confusion. In the latter instance, the child develops equal suggestibility to the physical and to the emotional so that he can block out what he feels as discomfort or pain. At times, he may be capable of purposely misbehaving, simply to experience the absence of pain because that is pleasurable to him. If he misbehaves, he cannot be sure whether he will be punished or caressed, but if he is punished, he can simply turn off the pain and, thereby, experience pleasure.

When children first go to school and interact with their peers, all the suggestibility conditioning from the mother comes to a head, and their suggestible behavior becomes more defined and exaggerated. Since all children of school age are concerned only with how *they* feel, and are not interested in trying to understand other children, each child is forced to retreat into the behavior that is most comfortable and least painful or uncomfortable to him.

Before entering school, the Physical children learned a behavior pattern of running headlong into the discipline, in order to get it over with so that they could have the gratification of the physical touch and attention that followed. They may even have purposely done something wrong, in order to get attention. They continue this pattern in school; and even if their attempts to obtain attention are rejected, they will continue to try, and their need for physical acceptance will become even more exaggerated.

The outgoing and aggressive behavior of the Physically suggestible children will cause the Emotionals to withdraw even more behind the defense of their emotions, so as to avoid any unpleasantness from a confrontation with the other children or the teacher. They also defend against any possible rejection or punishment that might result from any outward solicitation for closeness or intimacy. They avoid anything that will draw attention to their physical bodies because they are more comfortable with their emotions than with their physical capabilities.

In adulthood, a person's suggestibility is usually in constant change within the ranges of his predominant area of suggestibility.

It rarely changes from Physical to Emotional or vice versa, unless therapeutic intervention takes place. Suggestibility remains constant, only if a person ceases to expand, change, learn or relearn. In the hypnotic state, however, suggestibility can be altered because hypnosis is a regressed state. If the therapist communicates properly with the subject and creates the proper association with the subordinate suggestibility, a balanced condition is possible. Many times, suggestibility will alter itself during the course of therapy, as learning and expansion take place.

As we begin to understand how suggestibility is learned, we can understand how emotional and physical problems are learned. If we accept the premise that most problems are learned and that our suggestibility is the *how* and the *why* we learn, then it follows that most of our problems are caused by suggestibility. In hypnotherapy, we deal with how an undesired behavior can be unlearned and how a desired one can be learned to replace it. Hypnosis is our tool, and with it, we can affect the suggestibility of our clients through regression, desensitization, assertive or aversive therapy, and many other techniques. It is for this reason that the modern hypnotist is most appropriately called a *Suggestibility Behaviorist*.

## DOMINANT LAWS OF SUGGESTIBILITY

Successful therapeutic application of the theory of Emotional and Physical suggestibility requires an understanding of five dominant laws of suggestibility:

1. *The Law of Reverse Reaction*
2. *The Law of Repetition*
3. *The Law of Dominance*
4. *The Law of Delayed Action*
5. *The Law of Association*

Proper application of these laws will help you to utilize man's natural suggestibility to its fullest, by influencing him to respond to suggestions to a heightened degree. It is man's inclination toward two emotions – fear and greed – that makes him so susceptible to the influence of these laws. Because fear suppresses the ability to make a decision, any decision made for us during a fear reaction becomes the road of least resistance, and is readily accepted. Greed brings about a feeling of urgency and causes us to react without logical thinking.

Both, fear and greed are major tools used to the advantage of the advertiser in successful advertising. They are the prime forces motivating sales companies. On the other hand, our lawmakers design laws to combat unscrupulous people, who take advantage of us by capitalizing on our tendency toward fear and greed. As we discuss the dominant laws of suggestibility, keep in mind the relationship that fear and greed have to each of them.

The most commonly used law is the *Law of Reverse Reaction*, also called Reverse Psychology. It is used in personal, family, and business situations, as well as in all forms of advertising, and may have either negative or positive connotations. It can be used with all types of suggestions, including command, misdirection, confusion, persuasion, and passive suggestion. The reversal is especially potent because it reaches both critical and primitive areas of mind. For instance, it allows the subject a way out, if he is critical of a command, and also reinforces the command, if he desires it.

The law, simply stated, is that a person will respond to the stronger part of a suggestion, if the alternative is presented as considerably weaker. For example, in the eye challenge test, the dominant suggestions are, "Your eyes are stuck. You cannot open them. The harder you try, the tighter they become." The subject may *try* to open his eyes (weaker suggestion), but *cannot* (stronger suggestion). This is the reverse reaction. It is the same principle of reverse psychology that we see when a child is told he cannot do something. If doing it is more dominant, that is, gives greater pleasure than not doing it, the child will do it. Whenever the fear of missing something that gives pleasure or satisfies the ego (greed) is greater than the punishment that results from doing it, the subject will reverse the suggestions not to do it.

The *Law of Repetition* is illustrated by the fact that we constantly condition our minds and bodies to adapt to certain situations. If, for instance, we start playing handball once a week, in the beginning, our muscles tighten and hurt and our body feels weak after playing. With practice and conditioning, however, we gain strength and agility. When we enroll in a class to learn a new subject, we feel insignificant and mentally weak; but with constant repetition, we develop the habit of learning, and begin to react subconsciously without any conscious insecurity. Repetition of suggestions in hypnosis reinforces the new conditions, until they become subconscious habits.

The *Law of Dominance* can be described as a command position and can be applied to all the other laws because of its authoritarian structure. An example of the Law of Dominance is the suggestion of *deep sleep*. These words, usually spoken in an authoritative tone, represent a command, even if the induction up to that point has been maternal. The hypnotist assumes that the subject will, in fact, enter a deep sleep, and this becomes a dominant thought that the subject will accept without question.

The Law of Dominance also represents the dominant approach used in some instances by the therapist in inductions where he becomes the authoritative figure, such as, father, teacher, or boss, or gives the impression of being unreachable and all-knowing. This is a very effective therapeutic approach for certain clients who are in search of a dominant personality to guide them. It becomes a type of temporary transference that the hypnotist utilizes until the coping ability and decision-making ability of the client are improved.

The *Law of Delayed Action* is that when a suggestive idea is inferred, the subject will react to it whenever a jogging condition or situation that has been used in the original suggestive idea presents itself. Because an inference penetrates the subconscious mind slowly, due to its being unknown to the critical area of mind, it usually takes a day, two days, or even a week, before a reaction takes place. For example, if a subject is told to visualize himself in a situation where he is talking to his boss very confidently, and his boss has acknowledged by his actions that he sees this confidence, that particular suggestion will remain in the mind of the subject until he lives out the situation he has created by his visualization in hypnosis. He may even lack confidence until he has to face the real situation (i.e., seeing his boss); but once he has, the suggestions of confidence will take hold.

One of the notable characteristics of Emotionally suggestible people is their tendency to have delayed responses to inferred suggestions. As a rule, a generalization does not work well with an Emotionally suggestible subject. For this reason, a specific suggestion must be given. Delayed action suggestions have been know to cause a reaction as long as a year after they were given.

Once expectation has been created in a hypnotized subject, the *Law of Association* can be effectively put to use. This law simply indicates that whenever we repeatedly respond to one particular stimulus in the presence of another stimulus, we will soon begin to associate the one with the other. Then, whenever either stimulus is present, the other is recalled. A good example is that of a person who is always hypnotized in the same chair. After a while, he will associate that particular chair with hypnosis, and will enter the state the moment he sits in it – even without an induction. Another example is that of a subject hypnotized by the same operator over and over again. The voice of the hypnotist ultimately becomes associated with the hypnotic state; and, many times, the subject will respond to the voice of the hypnotist even more rapidly than to a post-suggestion to re-hypnosis. The Law of Association also refers to the tendency of a subject to respond to extraverbal movements and actions that indicate authority, confidence, or a position of control.

Another application of the Law of Association is that, if a subject accepts a first suggestion, he will accept the second suggestion also. Successful salespeople make use of this law each time they face a new client. If they can get the sales prospect to agree to a series of aspects of their sales talk, the next suggestion (asking for the order) will stand a very good chance of success. This concept deals with *knowns* and *unknowns*. Known suggestions are those that the subject or sales prospect has already experienced and can relate to as facts, thereby giving him a basis for the acceptance of subsequent unknown suggestions.

Reinforcing the Law of Association over and over again will increase the probability of its effectiveness. This is how the post-suggestion to re-hypnosis works. The subject has been given many associated suggestions with repetition, in order to arrive at the end result, which is *deep sleep*. Later, when the words *deep sleep* are used, he immediately associates the words with the previous conditioning – a known fact – and reacts without critical mind and enters the hypnotic state.

## LITERAL AND INFERRED SUGGESTIONS IN THERAPY

Hypnotherapy follows a basic pattern; and keeping this model in mind can be most helpful when you are shaping the therapeutic hour. During the initial phase of the session, the undesired behavior is examined and the client is allowed to guide the focus of the discussion. Remember, however, that this discussion will not vent out the negative events and will not create the more desirable behaviors. Venting or neutralizing can occur only when the consciousness is in abeyance, as in sleep or hypnosis.

Following the discussion of the unwanted behavior, the therapist brings up one or many positive alternatives to the unwanted behavior. In this way, the conscious mind is filled with considerations about the unwanted behavior and positive responses to it. The client is then hypnotized. This frees the conscious material to enter the critical area as positives and closes the door to negatives. If a client has been prepared properly, the message units that drop into his modern memory area are positive and the negatives are vented.

The reason a person feels so relaxed, light, and relieved when he comes out of the hypnotic state is that the critical area of his mind has dropped message units into the subconscious mind, and his negatives have been replaced by positives. The dreams that the client has following the session, whether he remembers them or not, will vent out remaining negatives. Keep this model of a therapy session in mind, as you continue with the material on the therapeutic use of literal and inferred suggestions.

The dynamics of a suggestion taking hold are virtually

identical with both Emotional and Physical subjects because both the predominantly Emotional and the predominantly Physical subjects have some of the opposite suggestibility, too. The Physically suggestible subject, however, manifests more visible physical responses than the Emotional subject.

The difference in suggestible traits is based on how we consciously take in a message, then on how our body responds to it. With the Physical, a single message unit is taken in literally as a thought, which becomes an image, then a physical feeling, and, finally, an emotional response. With the Emotional, on the other hand, a message unit is taken in as a thought, which then becomes an image, followed by an emotional feeling, and, ultimately, a physical reaction. This learning process begins with the conditioning toward *pain vs. pleasure,* mentioned earlier. The Physical literally seeks out pleasure and avoids pain; the Emotional functions on an inference and anticipates pain in search of pleasure. With a Physically suggestible subject, you work on the conflict literally; with an Emotionally suggestible subject, you work on what the conflict deprives him of. In both cases, the suggestions must be triggered back out of the mind by the environment.

If a Physically suggestible subject says, "I lack confidence in talking to people in a group situation," the suggestions you give are, "You will be confident talking to people in a group situation because it gives you pleasure," or, "you will be confident talking to people in a group situation because it allows you to become more successful." The clue is to give the suggestion literally (as the subject expressed it) and then to add positive reasons why he will have confidence. When he faces a group situation that in the past would have made him feel uncomfortable, the suggestion immediately shoots into the consciousness as a symbol. This symbol represents feeling, and the subject feels good about it, either physically or emotionally.

If an Emotionally suggestible subject says to you, "I lack confidence in talking to people in a group situation," your clue to the method of suggestion lies in finding out how he does feel in a group situation. He might feel inadequate, embarrassed, inferior, etc. Then hypnotize him, have him imagine himself feeling comfortable in a group situation (*systematic desensitization*), and suggest to him that he is an adequate, effective person and that embarrassment or inferiority or inadequacy will dissipate because he is comfortable. The suggestion takes away the pain and gives him pleasure. What it implies is that he is confident in a group setting. The clue to how to phrase suggestion to an Emotional subject lies in how he feels in a group situation, not the fact that he is lacking confidence. In other words, you must work with the inference that is affecting him.

The critical area of mind deals with knowns and unknowns; the conscious mind deals with literal and inferred interpretations. When a suggestion goes into the conscious mind and the consciousness goes into abeyance as a result of the hypnotic state, it has neither the chance to interpret nor the desire to fight the suggestion. Accordingly, the conscious mind allows the suggestion to go into the critical area and drop through without any analysis into the modern memory area of the subconscious mind.

Am Emotionally suggestible subject may be told that he is adequate. The next day in the waking state, that subject may face a situation where, in the past, he lacked confidence and felt inadequate. The suggestion then triggers from the modern memory area, through the critical area, and into the conscious mind, at which time the subject reacts, feeling more confident and adequate. Since he was not consciously aware of feeing inadequate, but just felt a lack of confidence, it might take a day or so or another even to make him realize that he is feeling more adequate and confident. This is an example of the *Law of Delayed Action*, particularly noticeable among subjects with Emotional suggestibility.

What is known to the critical area of mind of an Emotionally suggestible subject may be totally unknown to his consciousness, so the critical area is usually dealing with the effects of the word and not the actual word. If you suggest, "You are confident," the critical area may take that as an unknown and try to discard it. Then, when the individual actually faces the group situation, he may still feel uncomfortable because nothing has happened (the word confidence does not mean anything to him). He understands only what lack of confidence deprives him of, and it simply reminds him that he is deprived. However, if suggestions for lack of deprivation were added into the main suggestion, they would produce a positive response.

As mentioned earlier, there is a sub-category of Emotional suggestibility, called *intellectual suggestibility*. The best type of suggestion for a subject of this type are *persuasive, inferred suggestions*. For example:

> *"You are confident. Is it because I suggested it to you, or is it because you learned to become confident?"*

Since the suggestion, "You are confident," is literal, the Intellectual subject will disregard it immediately. But if he takes the two alternatives and tries to analyze which reason is correct, he has already accepted the inference that he is confident. Even if he comes to the conclusion that neither of the reasons applies and chooses another reason, he is still accepting the suggestion of confidence.

Another example would be:

> *"Why are you happy? Is it because I suggested it to you, or is it because I gave you a series of alternatives before we went into hypnosis?"*

Persuasive, inferred suggestions also work well with restricted Emotionals, who are afraid to respond to your suggestions because they feel threatened by you.

Working with Emotional suggestibility is much more involved than working with Physical suggestibility. Emotionally suggestible people represent at least 60% of all those in therapy; and if we look at it objectively, we will see that this is because most conflicts are created by Emotional suggestibility. Even those whose suggestibility is predominantly Physical will find that their emotional conflicts are caused by their Emotional suggestibility. A good rule of thumb to follow is: if Emotional suggestibility created the problem, Emotional suggestibility must be used to remove it; if Physical suggestibility created the problem, Physical suggestibility must be used to remove it.

Following are some of the common problems for which the two suggestibility types will come into therapy:

| **Physically Suggestible Subjects** | **Emotionally Suggestible Subjects** |
|---|---|
| Psychosomatic internal problems | Psychosomatic external physical physical problems |
| Fear of flying | Depression |
| Fear of heights | Anxieties |
| Fear of closed places | Indecisiveness |
| Procrastination | Male and female sexual problems |
| Sales motivation | Lack of confidence |
| Anxiety over exams | Fear of contamination |
| Rejections | Fear of death |
| Lack of confidence | Fear of loss of control |
| | Obsessive-compulsive behavior |
| | Hysterical conversions |

In general, the Emotional subjects suffer from more neurotic problems than do the Physicals. As a hypnotherapist, I believe that it is necessary to put more effort into understanding what Emotional suggestibility is, how it is created, and how one's receptiveness creates conflicts and problems. In turn, this increased effort can help us to understand how to remove these conflicts and problems from those who seek our help.

# INTRODUCTION TO
# SUGGESTIBILITY QUESTIONNAIRES

The suggestibility questionnaires that follow are the culmination of many years of therapy experience, examining the suggestibility of countless individuals. In order to construct the questionnaires, I initially included the most extreme suggestible traits characteristic of Physical or Emotional suggestibility. To these I added other suggestible traits, which are less obviously characteristic, yet still indicate an individual's suggestibility. In order to see how the written questionnaire compared with actual performance tests in the therapeutic setting, I gave subjects the performance tests and followed this by administering the questionnaires. The questionnaires were continually revised, until their scores consistently approximated the performance scores of hypnotic subjects.

The suggestibility questionnaires were created to be objective instruments, whereby any examiner can reproduce any other examiner's results with any particular subject. The questionnaires can actually eliminate the need for performance testing, but should not be used for this purpose because suggestibility can be influenced by such things as lack of good rapport with the operator, drug intake, or interpersonal conflicts with the operator. By comparing the performance testing with the questionnaire results, you can identify these situations, since their presence will lead to gross differences in scores. Also, the performance tests help to establish rapport and, for that reason alone, should not be replaced by the questionnaires.

Questions on both of the following suggestibility questionnaires must be answered before scoring.

# SUGGESTIBILITY QUESTIONNAIRE #1

1. Have you ever walked in your sleep during your adult life?  Yes  No

2. As a teenager, did you feel comfortable expressing your feelings to one or both of your parents?  Yes  No

3. Do you have a tendency to look directly into people's eyes and/or move closer to them, when discussing an interesting subject?  Yes  No

4. Do you feel most people you meet for the first time are uncritical of your appearance?  Yes  No

5. In a group situation with people you have just met, would you feel comfortable drawing attention to yourself, by initiating a conversation?  Yes  No

6. Do you feel comfortable holding hands or hugging someone you are in a relationship with, while other people are present?  Yes  No

7. When someone talks about feeling warm physically, do you begin to feel warm also?  Yes  No

8. Do you occasionally have a tendency to tune out, when someone is talking to you, and at times not even hear what the other person is saying because you are anxious to come up with your side of it?  Yes  No

9. Do you feel that you learn and comprehend better by seeing and/or reading, rather than hearing?  Yes  No

10. In a new class or lecture situation, do you usually feel comfortable asking questions in front of the group?  Yes  No

11. When expressing your ideas, do you find it important to relate all the details leading up to the subject, so the other person can understand it completely?  Yes  No

12. Do you enjoy relating to children?  Yes  No

13. Do you find it easy to be at ease and comfortable with your body movements, even when faced with unfamiliar people and circumstances?       Yes   No

14. Do you prefer reading fiction, rather than non-fiction?       Yes   No

15. If you were to imagine sucking on a sour bitter, juicy, yellow, lemon, would your mouth water?       Yes   No

16. If you feel that you deserve to be complimented for something well done, do you feel comfortable if the compliment is given to you in front of other people?       Yes   No

17. Do you feel that you are a good conversationalist?       Yes   No

18. Do you feel comfortable when complimentary attention is drawn to your physical body or appearance?       Yes   No

# SUGGESTIBILITY QUESTIONNAIRE #2

1. Have you ever awakened in the middle of the night and felt that you could not move your body and/or could not talk?  Yes  No

2. As a child, did you feel that you were more affected by the tone of voice of your parents than by what they actually said?  Yes  No

3. If someone you are associated with talks about a fear that you too have experienced, do you have a tendency to have an apprehensive or fearful feeling, as well?  Yes  No

4. If you are involved in an argument with someone, after the argument is over, do you have a tendency to dwell on what you could or should have said?  Yes  No

5. Do you have a tendency to tune out occasionally, when someone is talking to you – perhaps not even hear what was said – because your mind has drifted to something totally unrelated?  Yes  No

6. Do you sometimes desire to be complimented for a job well done, but feel embarrassed or uncomfortable when complimented?  Yes  No

7. Do you often have a fear or dread of not being able to carry on a conversation with someone you have just met?  Yes  No

8. Do you feel self-conscious, when attention is drawn to your physical body or appearance?  Yes  No

9. If you had your choice, would you rather avoid being around children most of the time?  Yes  No

10. Do you feel that you are not relaxed or loose in your body movements, especially when faced with unfamiliar people or circumstances?  Yes  No

11. Do you prefer reading non-fiction, rather than fiction?  Yes  No

12. If someone describes a very bitter taste, do you have difficulty experiencing the physical feeling of it?        Yes   No

13. Do you generally feel that you see yourself less favorably than others see you?        Yes   No

14. Do you tend to feel awkward or self-conscious initiating touch (holding hands, kissing, etc.) with someone you are in a relationship with, while other people are present?        Yes   No

15. In a new class or lecture situation, do you usually feel uncomfortable asking questions in front of the group, even though you may desire further explanation?        Yes   No

16. Do you feel uneasy, if someone you have just met looks you directly in the eyes when talking to you, especially if the conversation is about you?        Yes   No

17. In a group situation with people you have just met, would you feel uncomfortable drawing attention to yourself by initiating a conversation?        Yes   No

18. If you are in a relationship or are very close to someone, do you find it difficult or embarrassing to verbalize your love for him or her?        Yes   No

# SCORING INSTRUCTIONS FOR SUGGESTIBILITY QUESTIONNAIRES

1. Count the number of yes answers on Questionnaire #1. Give yourself five points for each **Yes** answer to Questions 3-18 and ten points for each **Yes** answer to Questions 1 and 2.

2. Do the same for Questionnaire #2.

3. Add the two scores together to obtain the combined score.

4. Locate your combined score number on the top horizontal line of the graph.

5. Locate the number that corresponds to your score for Questionnaire #1 on the far left vertical column of the graph.

6. Draw a horizontal line across the page from the 1 score; then draw a vertical line down from the combined score.

7. The number in the box where the two lines intersect is the adjusted percentile score for Questionnaire #1. It indicates your percentage of Physical Suggestibility.

8. Subtract that score from 100 to determine your percentage of Emotional Suggestibility.

## SCORE #1

*COMBINED SCORE #1 AND #2* (right-hand column)

| 0 | 5 | 10 | 15 | 20 | 25 | 30 | 35 | 40 | 45 | 50 | 55 | 60 | 65 | 70 | 75 | 80 | 85 | 90 | 95 | 100 | Combined |
|---|---|----|----|----|----|----|----|----|----|----|----|----|----|----|----|----|----|----|----|-----|----------|
| 0 | 10 | 20 | 30 | 40 | 50 | 60 | 70 | 80 | 90 | 100 |  |  |  |  |  |  |  |  |  |  | 50 |
| 0 | 9 | 18 | 27 | 36 | 45 | 55 | 64 | 73 | 82 | 91 | 100 |  |  |  |  |  |  |  |  |  | 55 |
| 0 | 8 | 17 | 25 | 33 | 42 | 50 | 58 | 67 | 75 | 83 | 92 | 100 |  |  |  |  |  |  |  |  | 60 |
| 0 | 8 | 15 | 23 | 31 | 38 | 46 | 54 | 62 | 69 | 77 | 85 | 92 | 100 |  |  |  |  |  |  |  | 65 |
| 0 | 7 | 14 | 21 | 29 | 36 | 43 | 50 | 57 | 64 | 71 | 79 | 86 | 93 | 100 |  |  |  |  |  |  | 70 |
| 0 | 7 | 13 | 20 | 27 | 33 | 40 | 47 | 53 | 60 | 67 | 73 | 80 | 87 | 93 | 100 |  |  |  |  |  | 75 |
| 0 | 6 | 13 | 19 | 25 | 31 | 38 | 44 | 50 | 56 | 63 | 69 | 75 | 81 | 88 | 94 | 100 |  |  |  |  | 80 |
| 0 | 6 | 12 | 18 | 24 | 29 | 35 | 41 | 47 | 53 | 59 | 65 | 71 | 76 | 82 | 88 | 94 | 100 |  |  |  | 85 |
| 0 | 6 | 11 | 17 | 22 | 28 | 33 | 39 | 44 | 50 | 56 | 61 | 67 | 72 | 78 | 83 | 89 | 94 | 100 |  |  | 90 |
| 0 | 5 | 11 | 16 | 21 | 26 | 32 | 37 | 42 | 47 | 53 | 58 | 63 | 68 | 74 | 79 | 84 | 89 | 95 | 100 |  | 95 |
| 0 | 5 | 10 | 15 | 20 | 25 | 30 | 35 | 40 | 45 | 50 | 55 | 60 | 65 | 70 | 75 | 80 | 85 | 90 | 95 | 100 | 100 |
| 0 | 5 | 10 | 14 | 19 | 24 | 29 | 33 | 38 | 43 | 48 | 52 | 57 | 62 | 67 | 71 | 76 | 81 | 86 | 90 | 95 | 105 |
| 0 | 5 | 9 | 14 | 18 | 23 | 27 | 32 | 36 | 41 | 45 | 50 | 55 | 59 | 64 | 68 | 73 | 77 | 82 | 86 | 91 | 110 |
| 0 | 4 | 9 | 13 | 17 | 22 | 26 | 30 | 35 | 39 | 43 | 48 | 52 | 57 | 61 | 65 | 70 | 74 | 78 | 83 | 87 | 115 |
| 0 | 4 | 8 | 13 | 17 | 21 | 25 | 29 | 33 | 38 | 42 | 46 | 50 | 54 | 58 | 63 | 67 | 71 | 75 | 79 | 83 | 120 |
| 0 | 4 | 8 | 12 | 16 | 20 | 24 | 28 | 32 | 36 | 40 | 44 | 48 | 52 | 56 | 60 | 64 | 68 | 72 | 76 | 80 | 125 |
| 0 | 4 | 8 | 12 | 15 | 19 | 23 | 27 | 31 | 35 | 38 | 42 | 46 | 50 | 54 | 58 | 62 | 65 | 69 | 73 | 77 | 130 |
| 0 | 4 | 7 | 11 | 15 | 19 | 22 | 26 | 30 | 33 | 37 | 41 | 44 | 48 | 52 | 56 | 59 | 63 | 67 | 70 | 74 | 135 |
| 0 | 4 | 7 | 11 | 14 | 18 | 21 | 25 | 29 | 32 | 36 | 39 | 43 | 46 | 50 | 54 | 57 | 61 | 64 | 68 | 71 | 140 |
| 0 | 3 | 7 | 10 | 14 | 17 | 21 | 24 | 28 | 31 | 34 | 38 | 41 | 45 | 48 | 52 | 55 | 59 | 62 | 66 | 69 | 145 |
| 0 | 3 | 7 | 10 | 13 | 17 | 20 | 23 | 27 | 30 | 33 | 37 | 40 | 43 | 47 | 50 | 53 | 57 | 60 | 63 | 67 | 150 |
| 0 | 3 | 6 | 10 | 13 | 16 | 19 | 23 | 26 | 29 | 32 | 35 | 39 | 42 | 45 | 49 | 52 | 55 | 58 | 61 | 65 | 155 |
| 0 | 3 | 6 | 9 | 13 | 16 | 19 | 22 | 25 | 28 | 31 | 34 | 38 | 41 | 44 | 47 | 50 | 53 | 56 | 59 | 63 | 160 |
| 0 | 3 | 6 | 9 | 12 | 15 | 18 | 21 | 24 | 27 | 30 | 33 | 36 | 39 | 43 | 45 | 48 | 52 | 55 | 58 | 61 | 165 |
| 0 | 3 | 6 | 9 | 12 | 15 | 18 | 21 | 24 | 26 | 29 | 32 | 35 | 38 | 42 | 44 | 47 | 50 | 53 | 56 | 59 | 170 |
| 0 | 3 | 6 | 9 | 11 | 14 | 17 | 20 | 23 | 26 | 29 | 31 | 34 | 37 | 41 | 43 | 46 | 49 | 51 | 54 | 57 | 175 |
| 0 | 3 | 6 | 8 | 11 | 14 | 17 | 19 | 22 | 25 | 28 | 31 | 33 | 36 | 39 | 42 | 44 | 47 | 50 | 53 | 56 | 180 |
| 0 | 3 | 5 | 8 | 11 | 14 | 16 | 19 | 22 | 24 | 27 | 30 | 32 | 35 | 38 | 41 | 43 | 46 | 49 | 51 | 54 | 185 |
| 0 | 3 | 5 | 8 | 11 | 13 | 16 | 18 | 21 | 24 | 26 | 29 | 32 | 34 | 37 | 39 | 42 | 45 | 47 | 50 | 53 | 190 |
| 0 | 3 | 5 | 8 | 10 | 13 | 15 | 18 | 21 | 23 | 26 | 28 | 31 | 33 | 36 | 38 | 41 | 44 | 46 | 49 | 51 | 195 |
| 0 | 3 | 5 | 8 | 10 | 13 | 15 | 18 | 20 | 23 | 25 | 28 | 30 | 33 | 35 | 38 | 40 | 43 | 46 | 48 | 50 | 200 |

*This page intentionally left blank.*

# CHAPTER 3 – HYPNOTIC INDUCTIONS

# THE INITIAL HYPNOTIC INDUCTION

There are four major steps that should comprise your initial hypnotic induction with a new client:

1) *The pre-induction*

2) *The conversion to hypnosis*

3) *The post-suggestion to re-hypnosis*

4) *The awakening procedure*

Most people know very little about hypnosis and tend to have preconceived ideas from reading books on the subject or from seeing a stage demonstration. The *pre-induction* is an introductory explanation of hypnosis. Its purpose is to dispel any preconceived ideas or fears that the subject may have about hypnosis and to give you the opportunity to give the subject suggestive ideas about how he will react and what he will experience in the state. It can also be carried through and used as an induction. The pre-induction should be geared to the specific problem with which you will be working, as well as to the suggestive pattern you intend to use after the induction.

For instance, if you have a new client who expresses a desire to gain confidence in certain areas of his life, you would give the following pre-induction:

*Hypnosis is a tool used to create suggestibility in the mind, allowing the individual to rid himself of inhibitions that may hold him back in life. Hypnosis also allows the individual to relax. In the process, tensions and pressures of the day will start to disappear. Through hypnosis, concentration and mental alertness are heightened. You are never unconscious or in a sleep state when you are hypnotized. Instead, you are more alert mentally, and your senses are more acute. The sounds around you may seem louder than usual because your hearing becomes hypersensitive in the state of hypnosis.*

*Hypnosis is created by words. Words affect us to the point where they can make us angry or sleepy, or they can stimulate ego sensations in our body. We can feel heaviness or lightness, or extremes of heat or cold. Drowsiness and relaxation will often take place.*

Up to this point, you should be watching to see if the rhythm of your voice and the words you are using are affecting your subject in any way. If the eyelids waver every time you describe heaviness, drowsiness, or sleepiness, you can convert to hypnosis very rapidly. Also, try to recognize the significance of any physical movements the client makes. If, for instance, he is following your eyes or subconsciously imitating your physical movements (scratching, nodding your head, etc.), this is an indication of Physical suggestibility. With this knowledge, you can proceed to talk your subject into hypnosis in the following way:

*As a person enters hypnosis, certain physical changes begin to take place. You will notice your breathing becoming deep, gentle, and rhythmic. Your lips and throat will become dry, and you will have the urge to swallow.*

If these two changes take place, continue by saying:

*Your arms, legs, and entire body will begin to feel heavier, your head will begin to jerk down slightly, and your eyelids will begin to flutter or blink, as you feel the drowsy pulsation of approaching sleep.*

If the physical reactions are present as you talk, the client is ready to enter hypnosis. Your tone of voice should then change to a more direct and commanding tone, as you say:

*I will now count from five backwards to zero; and with each count, your eyelids will grow heavier and you will go deep asleep. Five...four...three...two...one...zero!*

Snap your fingers and say in a commanding voice:

*Deep sleep!*

In this way, the pre-induction speech itself is used, both to gauge the subject's suggestibility and to induce hypnosis. There are many other ways to address a subject's suggestibility and to convert to hypnosis. Several of these tests and conversions will be discussed in this chapter.

At one time or another, every hypnotist will have certain clients come into his office who say that they cannot be hypnotized because others have tried and failed. Almost without exception, these will be Emotionally suggestible subjects with whom the previous hypnotist used a literal, paternal induction. Because the subject's suggestibility is already obvious to you in this instance, testing is not necessary, and you can go right into a maternal pre-induction and conversion to hypnosis. The pre-induction should describe what an Emotional subject will feel while in the state of hypnosis. For instance, you might say:

> *Right now, you are concentrating on my voice, but when you enter the hypnotic state, you will not only be aware of my voice, but you will also hear sounds around you that seem to be louder than usual. Many thoughts of the day will pass through your mind, even questions as to whether or not you are actually hypnotized. You will feel physically relaxed, and you may feel some lightness, heaviness, or tingling in the body; but the important thing is that, even though these thoughts enter your mind, you will lose the desire to fight the suggestions that I am giving you because you really won't want to open your eyes or move out of the chair at that time.*

Because this subject is Emotionally suggestible, you would then proceed with an Emotional test conversion, such as, the inferred arm-raising conversion. Although this induction is geared to the extremely Emotionally suggestible subject, it is also effective with less extreme Emotionals and even with Physicals. It is not really a test, as is the regular arm-raising test, because it does not actually help to determine the subject's suggestibility, but merely utilizes the suggestibility that you already know is present. It cannot be ended simply with the test, but must follow through as a conversion to hypnosis.

*In a few moments, I am going to be testing your suggestibility. This is one test that you cannot fail, so you don't have to help me or hinder me. A series of physiological changes will take place, as well as some emotional changes. I will make you aware of everything that is going on, as it is happening.*

*Now, sit very straight in the chair, feet flat on the floor, left hand on your left leg and right hand on the table.*

The subject is now in the correct position for a regular arm-raising test. Once he is in this position, tell him:

*I want you to look directly at me, staring right into my eyes. Do not answer me verbally – just shake your head to indicate yes or no. If you do not know the answer, just keep staring. Let me try to find the answer.*

The reason you have the subject shake his head rather than talk is that talking would give him an opportunity to expand on more than the word *yes* or *no* and would also break the rhythmic pattern. Shaking the head also helps to disorganize the subject.

The purpose of the questions is to get six or seven yes answers. In order to insure that you will receive affirmative answers, ask questions from the Emotional suggestibility questionnaire. During this time, you should also question the subject to see if he has been on medication or drugs in the last twenty-four hours, since drugs will affect his reactions. Tranquilizing drugs suppress ego sensations and, thereby, alter responses to physical tests. Hypnotic drugs, such as, marijuana and cocaine will heighten ego sensations and make the subject appear more Physically suggestible than he really is.

The last question you ask the subject should be, Can you visualize with your eyes closed? If he says he can, have him close his eyes and visualize his right hand. If not, have him close his eyes and *imagine* his right hand.

Next, pick obvious physical reactions the subject will have and suggest that when he feels them taking place, he will nod his head yes. Since an Emotional functions on high expectation, the physical changes will be exaggerated. Now tell him that:

> *In a few moments, you will feel your concentration drawn to your breathing. When you feel you breathing change, nod your head yes. [Whenever the attention is drawn to the breathing, it will automatically expand.]*

> *Next, concentrate on your eyes. When you feel your eyes trying to roll upward under your eyelids, causing a movement in the eyelids, nod your head yes. When you become aware that you feel dryness in your lips and throat that may lead to swallowing, nod your head yes.*

> *Now, imagine that I am taking hold of your wrist, and I am pulling it up. When you begin to feel some tension or lifting in your wrist, nod your head yes. I'll be pulling your hand up in rhythm with every breath that you take in. When you feel this, nod your head yes, and the hand will continually lift and rise, going upward and inward toward your face, with every breath you take in.*

Use the word up only when the subject inhales. Continue this movement until the hand is about to touch the head, telling the subject that:

> *When your hand touches your head, you will reach the peak of your suggestibility and you will go into the hypnotic state upon skin contact between your hand and your head.*

All the physical changes mentioned above will occur naturally with a highly Emotionally suggestible subject, although he will be unaware of the changes, until you bring them to his attention. When the subject constantly nods his head, he not only infers that the reaction is going to take place, but he also forms a habit of following your suggestions. Suggesting physical changes as they are happening, and having the subject participate by nodding his head, will also remove any fear of loss of control, allowing the subject to enter a highly suggestible state right from the beginning, without any restrictions.

You are also using an inferred approach, when you increase the subject's expectation toward the hypnotic state by the pre-induction procedure of telling him that you are going to count from five backwards to zero, and that when you reach zero, he will enter the hypnotic state. However, if you touch his forehead as you are counting, the sudden touch will infer that he is already at zero, and will, therefore, trigger him into the hypnotic state, even before you reach zero.

Before awakening the subject, you must implant a post-suggestion to re-hypnosis. The following is a generalized post-suggestion that leave no room for doubt:

| | |
|---|---|
| *Each and every time* | Covers the present and the future. |
| *I suggest sleep to you* | The *I* and *you* are exaggerated. |
| *You will sleep* | All are exaggerated. |
| *Quickly, soundly, and deeply* | Exaggerate *deeply*, especially with a deep subject. |
| *And the physical body will be very relaxed.* | The subject is more prone to accepting the post-suggestion because it is beneficial and eliminates any possibility of threat. |

The first word of the post-suggestion that a subject hears can determine his entire reaction. For example, you could unknowingly destroy the effect of the suggestion, by saying, Now, each and every time … because the subject might interpret now as literally meaning now, during this session, at this moment only. The first sound always becomes the first apparent power word in a post-suggestion; so, unless you mean now, at this moment only, do not use that word in the post-suggestion to re-hypnosis.

Another example of power words and how they can affect a post-suggestion in certain instances is evidenced with extremely Physically suggestible subjects, who take suggestions very literally. It is always advisable to condition this type of subject to give his verbal consent to accept a post-suggestion. The reason for this is that, if you give a post-suggestion, such as, "Each time I touch your forehead, you will go deep asleep," a physically deep subject will accept this suggestion literally and will react to re-hypnosis, but he may also become overly suggestible in the future to anyone who claims to be I. Also, if someone catches him off-guard and touches his forehead, the subject may enter the hypnotic state and have an abreaction to the original acceptance of the suggestion. Even if the suggestion works, depth may be impaired. To prevent any undesired reactions, the operator should allow the subject to express his own will. After the hypnotist receives consent, he should reword the post-suggestion, as follows:

*Each and every time I suggest sleep to you and have your verbal consent, then, and only then, will you sleep quickly, soundly, and deeply.*

Following, is an example of a misdirective, or inferred post-suggestion, to re-hypnosis, to be used with Emotionally suggestible subjects:

*You entered the state of hypnosis, when I touched your forehead, and you have continually gone deeper. Each time I suggest sleep to you, you enter more quickly because you are becoming accustomed to it.*

The inference is that, the next time you touch his forehead, the suggestion to re-hypnosis will be activated. Now, a conditioned association has taken place. It will become even stronger, if reactional hypnosis (awakening the subject and re-hypnotizing him with a post-suggestion over and over) is used.

If a post-suggestion fails, we can safely assume one of three things: that the post-suggestion was not completely understood subconsciously by the subject, that the suggestion was too complicated to be followed in the depth attained, or that the post-suggestion depreciated and no longer affected the subject. The subject's conscious memory of the given post-suggestion is never a determinant of whether or not he will react to it.

Awakening the client at the end of the session is very easy, but very essential. Simply say:

*In a few moments, I will count upwards from zero to five. Five, as always, represents wide awake, physically relaxed, emotionally calm, and intellectually alert. Zero...one...two... three...four...five.... Wide awake! Wide awake!*

From this first session on, hypnotic conditioning is no longer necessary, although your therapy must always fit the subject's suggestibility. These initial steps prevent the operator from making the mistake of trying to push for depth, when depth will occur naturally, if the proper steps are taken.

The first induction is of paramount importance because it is the beginning from which all therapy will progress. If the client begins feeling improvement from the onset, the therapy is given a decisive, positive impetus. Always keep in mind that the main objectives of the first induction are to build expectation and imagination and to leave the subject with feelings of relaxation, well-being, and increased confidence in himself and the therapeutic process.

## SUGGESTIBILITY TESTS AND CONVERSIONS TO HYPNOSIS

Testing a subject's suggestibility has a two-fold purpose:

1) To determine the degree of Emotional and Physical Suggestibility.

2) To convert to hypnosis without the subject expecting it to happen, which prevents any possibility of him helping or hindering you.

You should always use direct, literal suggestion when testing either Physical or Emotional subjects for the first time, in order to determine where their suggestibility lies because a positive response to an inferred test does not necessarily prove Emotional suggestibility, as might be expected. The inference itself would affect the Emotional subject, but a Physical subject could interpret the inference literally and respond to the literal meaning. However, a response to physical tests does indicate Physical, rather than Emotional suggestibility and depth. Therefore, the degree of the lack of physical responses would reveal the degree of Emotional suggestibility.

The written suggestibility questionnaires indicate the pure potential of a person's suggestibility. If the proper induction is used and good rapport is built, the subject should reach the same suggestible depth indicated by his questionnaire. However, the subject may be blocked from reaching his potential depth in instances when the confidence or ability of the operator is lacking, an improper pre-induction or induction has been used, or when the subject is on medication or drugs. Consequently, performance tests should be given each time you see the subject until he reaches his potential depth because that is his most susceptible state.

All of the tests described in this chapter are carried through and used as hypnotic inductions, even though they can also be used simply as tests of suggestibility and ended before the conversion to hypnosis. The reason for this is that, when a subject responds to a physical test, it is advisable to continue with the conversion to hypnosis in order to utilize the suggestibility you have already created. Always give a post-suggestion to re-hypnosis before awakening the subject and suggest feelings of well-being as you awaken him.

If your subject does not respond to physical tests, you know he is Emotionally suggestible, and your methods from this point on should be maternal and inferred. *Maternalism*, a rhythmic, lulling patter, which coaxes, rather than commands a subject into the hypnotic state, is always the most effective approach to use with the Emotional subject. *Paternalism* is an authoritarian technique, using a rapid, commanding patter, and should be used only with Physically suggestible subjects. Even though a Physically suggestible subject will respond to both paternalism and maternalism, it is always preferable to begin with a maternal approach and then become more paternal once you have established rapport.

# FINGER-SPREADING TEST

After the subject is seated, tell him to place his feet flat on the floor and extend his hand out approximately twelve inches in front of his face, with the palm inward and the tip of the longest finger the same height as his nose. Tell him to concentrate on his fingers spreading, as you repeat the words, "fingers pulling, separating," over and over, until you see the fingers begin to spread. Suggest that the subject's hand and arm pull inward toward his face, "pulling, drawing, jerking inward." Continue to repeat the suggestion until his hand touches his face.

To convert from this test into hypnosis, suggest that, as his hand pulls inward, his eyelids will grow heavy and begin to close. When he feels skin contact, he will go deeply asleep. Snap your fingers, as the subject's hand touches his face, and say, Deep sleep! At this point, a challenge may be given:

> *Your hand is now stuck to your face, stuck tight, and you cannot pull it away. You may try, but the more you try, the tighter it sticks. You cannot pull your hand from your face.*

Wait a few moments, and then say:

> *Now, forget your hand and go deeper asleep.*

Take the subject's hand and tell him to relax it and that, as it moves down to his side, he will go deeper.

# HAND-CLASP TEST

Your subject can be in either a sitting or a standing position for the hand-clasp test. A sitting position is preferable, of course, if you plan to use the test as a conversion to hypnosis.

To begin, have the subject extend his arms straight out in front of him, with his elbows stiff and his fingers interlocked, and tell him to stare at one of his fingernails. Then tell him:

> *I will count from five down to zero, and with each count, you will feel your hands tightening and your fingers locking. When*

*I reach zero, your hands will be tightly clasped and your elbows locked, and you will not be able to open your hands.*

Continue in a paternal tone of voice:

*FIVE ... hands and fingers tightening. FOUR ... hands growing tighter and tighter. THREE ... hands very tight, still locking. TWO ... feel the pressure in your elbows, as they begin to lock ... ONE ... elbows locked, hands still tighter and tighter. ZERO ... hands and fingers tightly locked. You cannot open them. The harder you try, the tighter they stick.*

To convert to hypnosis, simply tell him:

*You cannot pull your hands apart. And now, your eyes are becoming heavy, eyelids are closing ... eyelids very heavy and closing.*

When you see his eyes close, say firmly:

*Tightly closed! And now, deep sleep!*

As you give this final suggestion, snap your fingers or clap your hands to jar the subject into the state.

## ARM-RAISING TEST

In my opinion, the arm-raising test is the most important technique for a hypnotist to master. Its tremendous value is attributable to the many advantages it has over other approaches – advantages for the hypnotist and subject alike. For example:

1. It offers a ready conversion into hypnosis.

2. It reaches the extremely Emotionally suggestible subjects, who have formerly been considered unhypnotizable.

3. It is an easy way for the hypnotist to demonstrate that the subject is capable of responding to suggestive ideas.

4. It is actually an exercise, not a test, so it cannot be failed. This reduces the subject's anxiety about doing the right thing, and keeps him from acting a particular way in order to please the operator.

5. It presents the operator with the opportunity to use misdirection, inferred suggestions, and literal suggestions – all in a natural way.

6. It provides an opportunity for the operator to increase the Physical or Emotional suggestibility of the subject, according to what he thinks is necessary for the ensuing therapy.

7. It is a good technique for hypnotists in training, since it requires no special equipment and is relatively easy to learn.

8. It can be used to hypnotize groups, as well as individuals.

There are two basic approaches to the arm-raising test. The first is used if the subject appears to respond readily. If the subject is slow to respond or is resistant, it may be necessary to employ the second approach.

**FIRST APPROACH:** Start with the pre-induction, in order to build rapport. At this point, the subject's eyes may be either open or closed. Use rhythmic speech and some misdirection, saying:

*I am going to test your suggestibility. Just sit back in your chair, feet flat on the floor, right hand and arm on the table. Concentrate on your wrist. Do not help or hinder me. Just imagine that everything I say is happening because it actually will happen. Many times, when you have been sleeping or just sitting relaxed, you have felt a jerk in the muscles of your hands, arm, or legs. This is a subconscious release or contraction of your involuntary muscles.*

Now, begin the patter:

*In a few moments, you will notice your right hand and arm, from your fingertips to your elbow, beginning to grow light and having a tendency to lift and rise ... up, up, rising ... jerking ... light as a feather. Now, imagine I have a string tied to your wrist, and I am pulling it up, up, higher and higher, lifting, rising ... higher and higher ... up, up, rising ... jerking ... light as a feather....*

Continue this patter and, if you see that the subject is pushing down and fighting you, add misdirection, by saying:

*Now, you begin to feel your head and your other hand and arm growing heavier. The left arm and hand are heavy. The right arm and hand lighter and lighter, up, up, light as a feather.*

When you see a twitch or movement, say:

*Now, your mind has accepted the suggestion, and your left arm is heavier … left hand heavier … right arm lighter and now lifting…*

Continue the patter, until the arm is at about a 45-degree angle, with the elbow still resting on the table. Then start adding more suggestions for confusion:

*Now you feel your right elbow pushing down, harder and harder. You cannot put your arm down, no matter how hard you try. You may try, but the more you try, the lighter and stiffer it becomes, for you feel the tightness in the forearm, as the elbow pushes down … arm still lighter and lighter, going up, up….*

Wait a few seconds, until the subject tries to put his arm down, and if he fails (which he will, if the patter is right and he has enough Physical suggestibility), begin to convert to hypnosis, again using the patter in a rhythmic tone:

*You will now begin to feel your hand twisting and turning at your wrist, and your fingers turning toward your face … twisting, turning … lifting, rising … up, up, higher and inward, feeling your hand and face drawing closer and closer, as if drawn together by magnetism … hand and face, closer and closer … twisting and turning … the hand drawing closer and closer, and the head moving down, down, closer to your hand … feeling your breathing becoming deep, gentle, and rhythmic … lips dry … throat dry … and the urge to swallow becomes prominent … and soon you will feel skin contact, as your hand touches your face.*

Continue the patter, until the hand just about touches the face. Then say:

*As the hand touches the face, you will go deep [snap fingers], deep asleep!*

At this point, issue a challenge, such as:

*Your eyelids are stuck tightly shut, and you cannot open them.*

or:

*Your hand is now stuck to your face, and you cannot move it away.*

An inferred arm-raising can be used with a highly Emotionally suggestible subject, whose arm will rise, if he concentrates on an outside object lifting it. For example, you might have him imagine that you are taking hold of his wrist and lifting it, or that a string holding a helium balloon is tied around his wrist, and as the balloon goes up, so will his hand and arm. Then proceed with the patter and conversion, as above.

**SECOND APPROACH:** If neither the literal nor the inferred version works, place the subject's right arm on the table with the elbow, forearm, and hand lying face down on the table. Continue as in the first approach. Should the arm come up very slowly or the subject resist because of defenses, you will notice that either the fingers are pushing down or the person is opening his eyes, talking to you, telling you it is not working, or finding some reason to distract you or himself from it. At that moment, tell him:

*Everything is fine. Now slide your hand forward, until the elbow is at least twelve inches in front of your body. Lift your wrist as high as you can without your fingers leaving the table. Press your fingers down on the table and press your elbow down very firmly, relaxing the wrist. Now stare at your fingers, and as you begin to see or feel your fingers move away from the table, close your eyes and experience the continuing upward movement of your arm.*

This second approach will work where the first has failed because the reluctant subject has been consciously or subconsciously fighting you and has created a tension in his wrist to hold the hand down. When the wrist is bent in this awkward position, the tendency of the muscles is to straighten the wrist out again, in order to alleviate the tension. Add to this the suggestion that he will feel his elbow pushing down, and the only natural reaction is for the hand and arm to go up. By this time, there have been so many message units poured into the subject's mind, the subconscious mind cannot analyze what is taking place, so the escape to hypnosis via the arm-raising conversion is welcomed.

The arm-raising test can also be done with the palm up, leaving the client nothing to hang onto. Since flight is a defense mechanism to protect against loss of control, this created loss of control will cause the subconscious to respond to the suggestion of hypnotic sleep, which represents flight.

## ARM-DRAWING AND SHOCK CONVERSION TEST

This induction is created through paternalism and shock command. It is a simple induction, and the subject is not supposed to know the mechanics.

Place the subject in an upright chair, with his feel flat on the floor and his arms extended outward, until his shoulders begin rounding out and coming forward. Then place your thumb on the inside of his wrists and hold his arms apart. (If you release his arms at this point, they will draw in by themselves.) Hold his arms in this position, while you tell him:

*In a moment, I will release your arms. Your hands and arms will pull inward, as if a force is drawing them together. When your hands touch, you will go deep asleep. Now, concentrate on my voice and look into my eyes [release his hands], as your hands and arms constantly draw closer and closer, drawing inward, pulling together.*

The expectation will build, as the arms pull in. Your hand should be placed on the outside of the subject's hands so that you can follow his hands without touching them. When his hands are about six to eight inches apart, push them together and command, "Deep sleep!" The sudden shock and the suggestion of sleep result in a very rapid conversion to hypnosis. Now suggest that his hands and arms will grow heavy, limp, loose, and relaxed. As his arms begin to drop down, release them, allowing them to fall in his lap, and say, "Deeper asleep!"

# FALLING-BACK TEST

When the falling back test is used for conversion into hypnosis, your approach should be commanding and paternal, and the subject must be unaware of what you are going to do. To begin, stand with one foot forward and the other securely behind you, in order to be sure you are sufficiently braced to catch the subject, as he falls backwards. The subject should stand upright with his feet placed close together, shoulders back, and head upward, looking directly at a spot on the ceiling. Place your hands on the subject's shoulders, pushing slightly forward and down. This pushing on the subject's shoulders has the effect of making him want to push backward and, thereby, unknowingly help you.

Then, in a soft, lulling, maternal voice, suggest:

*In a few moments, you will feel my hands lifting off your shoulders; and, as you do, you will feel me drawing you backwards. I will catch you, so just relax. Now concentrate on my voice.*

As your hands lift from his shoulders, say in a firm, commanding voice, "Back, back, falling back." As the subject starts to move, tell him that his eyes will now close, and he will feel himself beginning to fall back. Catch him as he falls and command, "Deep Sleep!" as you lower him slowly to the floor. At the time he is being lowered, give a post-suggestion to re-hypnosis and then awaken him.

# PROGRESSIVE RELAXATION INDUCTION

The *progressive relaxation* is an important secondary type of induction. It is secondary because an operator using the progressive will not be able to determine the subject's exact suggestibility, nor will he be able to take the subject to the exact depth desired. I sincerely believe that it is both therapeutically ineffective and an abdication of responsibility to use the progressive as the initial induction. However, many hypnotists persist in using it as such because they do not feel confident that the subject will respond to a conversion induction.

The progressive is most effective when used immediately following a conversion induction. While the subject is still in hypnosis, he is asked to open his eyes without awakening and to move to an adjacent recliner chair. The progressive is used and therapy follows. Because the subject is deeply relaxed and is in a still position, there are fewer body-to-brain message units, and his receptiveness to suggestions is increased. This maternal induction is equally effective with Emotional and Physical subjects, and is compatible with both inferred and literal suggestions.

The progressive relaxation induction can be used on an individual or a group. The basic procedure is to relax the various areas of the body, allow the subject(s) to remain still for approximately five minutes, then catch the mind off-guard and induce hypnosis. This secondary induction is a must for every hypnotist.

*Sit back in your chair. Uncross your legs. Close your eyes. Now begin breathing very deeply, taking five deep breaths; and with every breath you exhale, you will become more deeply relaxed.*

*After the fifth breath, concentrate on the weight of your shoes. Your shoes, being foreign to your normal body weight, will begin to fee heavy, and this heavy relaxation from your toes to your heels to your ankles will become very prominent. You are now feeling this heavy relaxation moving upward into the calves of your legs ... feeling the weight of your legs pushing down, heavier and heavier ... and feeling your legs relaxing deeply ... deeply relaxing ... and this heavy relaxation moves into the knees, as you concentrate only on my voice.*

*Pay no attention to any outside sounds, except my voice, for these outside sounds are everyday sounds of life and cannot distract or disturb you, but will tend to relax you and allow you to go even deeper into this deep, heavy relaxation.*

*Now, feel the relaxation moving upward into your thighs and hips and through the mid-section of your body ... feel the stomach muscles relaxing ... deeply relaxing ... and the entire chest area becomes saturated with relaxation. Breathing becomes very deep, gentle, and rhythmic, and the drowsy, sleepy, daydreaming feeling of relaxation takes over ... LETTING GO! ... drifting down, deeper and deeper, and your arms, hands, and fingers are relaxing ... feeling a numb, pleasant, tingling feeling through your fingers, as this relaxation grows deeper and deeper.*

*Neck muscles are relaxing and all the little muscles in the scalp are letting go, feeling as if the blood is circulating very close to the skin. This relaxation moves down over your forehead and down over your eyelids like a dark veil of sleep, as your jaw muscles relax deeply ... deeply relaxing ... and growing heavier.*

*And as I count from five down to zero, each count will represent deep relaxation, and you will feel the body relaxing even more and letting go ... deeper and deeper ... and when I reach zero, you will go deep asleep. Now, FIVE ... letting go ... FOUR ... THREE ... TWO ... ONE ... ZERO ... [snap your fingers] DEEP ASLEEP!*

Now, quickly misdirect the subject, by saying:

*Now concentrate on my voice, and you will go even deeper asleep with every breath that you exhale.*

Before awakening the subject, give suggestions for re-hypnosis and feelings of well-being and relaxation. Awaken him by reversing the count from zero to five.

## EYE FASCINATION INDUCTION

The eye fascination is one of the inductions most commonly over-used by the unsophisticated hypnotist. Its use should be limited to times when the subject's reactions give you a definite indication that it will work. For instance, if, when interviewing a client, you notice that his eyes have a tendency to fade or that his eyes are blinking or partially closing, it would give you a direct lead into this induction.

Seat the subject in an upright position in a chair with his hands in his lap. Tell him to stare straight ahead, looking directly into a particular object or light. Make sure his eyes are tipping slightly upward, in order to create fatigue of the eyes. Then begin to suggest rapidly and paternally that his eyelids are growing extremely heavy and that soon they will have a tendency to close. Tell him, "When your eyelids close, you will enter a deep hypnotic sleep."

Continue this pattern of stimulating heaviness of the eyelids, until you see them beginning to close, flutter, or flicker. At this time, you should be standing close to the subject, preferably at his side. Move your hand very rapidly to his forehead (without him seeing your hand) and touch him lightly with your finger, saying, "Deep Sleep!" At that moment, push his hands off his lap to create a limp, loose feeling in his body. Then continue with a deepening procedure.

## HYPNOSCOPE INDUCTION

A Hypnoscope is a small rotary motor encased in a box. It is equipped with a variety of detachable discs with varying patterns. As the disc spins, it creates an optical illusion effect. The Hypnoscope itself does not actually hypnotize the subject, but serves mainly to create fatigue of the eyes and disorganization of the brain patterns.

A typical approach using the Hypnoscope would be to have the subject sit in a position where he is looking slightly up at the disc and to suggest that:

*As you concentrate on this whirling, drawing effect, you will begin to feel yourself being drawn into this inner circle. You will begin to feel your eyelids being pulled down … feeling heaviness in the eyelids and distortion in your view, and the eyelids continually pull down, as you are drawn inward. Your arms, your legs, your entire body are being drawn down into a deeper and deeper state of relaxation and sleep. Your eyelids are heavy, and you feel you will begin to follow my count of five backwards to zero. With each count, your eyelids will become even heavier. Zero will represent deep sleep. Even after you enter the hypnotic sleep, you will see the image of that whirling disc.*

The count from five to zero should be timed to begin just as you see the fluttering of the eyelids beginning to close. The count should be in an authoritarian tone of voice. Zero should be louder than the other numbers, and the snap of the fingers should be timed with the words *zero* and *deep sleep*. Most subjects will have an after vision of the whirling disc for a few moments after their eyes are closed.

The Hypnoscope induction is useful with young adults, and especially children under the age of fifteen. It is not recommended for persons over forty years of age because the disorganization and the visual distortion could cause dizziness or even nausea in an older person.

## AUTO-DUAL METHOD

The *auto-dual method* is an approach to hypnosis that has been designed for the analytical or Intellectually suggestible subject. When a subject arranges to see a hypnotist, pays for a session, and then tries to analyze himself out of hypnosis, we can assume that he has a fear of being controlled by the operator. The auto-dual method prevents this type of individual from analyzing what the operator is saying or doing, thereby, causing him to enter the hypnotic state through a form of misdirection. It allows him to believe that he is hypnotizing himself, instead of being hypnotized by the operator. Although this is not actually the case, this method does break down resistance, allowing the operator to reach the subject more easily.

The mechanics of the auto-dual method are as follows: Place your subject in a straight-backed chair. Tell him to put his feet flat on the floor, to place his right index finger on the pulse of his left wrist, and to stare directly at the fingernail of his right index finger. He has now accepted three suggestions consciously, which prepares him to accept what follows. Now, have him repeat after you the following:

*I will now enter the state of hypnosis for the reasons of deep relaxation and self-control. I will count from five down to zero, and with each count, I will become more deeply relaxed. When I reach zero, I will go deep asleep. Five ... I begin to feel my breathing growing deep, gentle, and rhythmic.*

Suggest this just as his breathing pattern begins to vary. The subject himself is usually not aware of the natural change in his breathing, as he prepares to enter the hypnotic state. The tendency of his head to drop forward should also be utilized. The instant you see his head jerking forward, suggest that his head is growing heavy and is beginning to drop forward.

*Four ... I begin to feel heaviness in my eyelids, as I become drowsier and sleepier. [His eyelids will naturally tire from staring at his fingernail.] Three ... I begin to feel every muscle, nerve, and fiber in my body relaxing, deeply relaxing. Two ... My arms, my legs, my entire body, are now deeply relaxed. One ... My eyelids grow even heavier, my is breathing more rhythmic. I am deeply relaxed. Zero ... Deep asleep!*

The fact that the subject is talking and repeating after you, prevents him from simultaneously analyzing what is being said; so when you reach zero, he is psychologically and physically prepared to follow the final suggestion of deep, hypnotic sleep, in order to defend himself against his own fears of being controlled.

To awaken him, simply reverse the count and say, "Wide awake."

## CHILD INDUCTION

As a general rule, children are easy to hypnotize. Most of them are very deep subjects. You should use very little misdirection when working with children because they have a way of seeing beyond it. They are very literal, and many times, when you try to misdirect them, they will look not for what you try to make obvious, but for what they felt you meant. Using gadgets, crystal balls, flashing lights, or any fascination point, will work well with children, since they have a tendency to lack strong concentration. The key to hypnotizing children is to hold their concentration long enough to reach them.

The most effective approach is as follows: Have the child sit in an upright chair. Choose a point of fascination for him to stare at, such as a crystal ball or penlight, and hold it above the child's forehead, as you stand to one side of him. Place your other hand on the back of his head and neck and move him from side to side, going first away from you and then slowly back. Hold the crystal ball or penlight in place. (If you move it, the child's attention might be drawn to something else in the room.) As the child is moved from side to side, he is able to feel his body beginning to relax, and he loses his resistance, as he becomes loose and limp.

When you feel the child going into hypnosis, suggest that his eyes feel sleepy and that his eyelids are growing heavy. Then, when his eyes crystallize and eyelids blink, bring the ball or penlight down to touch his forehead, and say:

*You will feel the ball [or light] touch your head and, as it does, you will go deep asleep, always hearing my voice.*

Touch his head about the same time as his eyes close, and say, "Deep asleep!" Then tell him:

*Your body is so heavy that you will become limp and loose, just like a rag doll.*

Tell him that you are going to lift him out of the chair and put him into a more comfortable one, and when you lift him, he will feel a heavy, limp, loose feeling all through his body and will go even deeper asleep.

When working with a child, it is always a good policy to ask him as you go along if he understands what you have said. Have him nod his head, if he does. If you tell him just before you hypnotize him that you are going to do this, he will become very receptive to you. When you are giving him a suggestion, ask him if he wants to accept it. Get him to cooperate with you, as if you are working together. Play it as a game. You can joke, laugh, and talk to him, as if you were a child. You have to move into his age level and act like him for him to respond most effectively to you and to the therapy.

## ANALYSIS OF INDUCTION

The analysis of induction chart that follows allows you to make important notes on a subject so that, as sessions progress, you can remember and continue to use the most effective approach for that particular individual. It also shows you the pattern of change taking place with your client from session to session.

**Name of Subject:** _____

**Date:** _____

**Attitude of Subject:**      Calm _____     Fearful _____
                            Nervous _____ Indifferent _____

**Type of Induction Used:**

**Induction Timing:**      Perfect _____    Too Slow _____
                            Too Fast _____

**Physical Movements:**     Lazy _____    Deliberate _____
**During Induction:**         Unnoticeable _____

**Subject's Suggesitibility:**

**Subject's Comfort:**      Reaction to Distance _____

                           Reaction to Closeness _____

                           Reaction to Touch _____

                           Reaction to Maternalism _____

                           Reaction to Paternalism _____

**Physical Behavior:**      Total Relaxation (letting go) _____

**While in the Hypnotic State:**

                           Erratic Abreactional _____

                           Movements (fear) _____

                           Constant Body Movements (mistrust) _____

                           Other _____

                           _____

**Post Suggestion to Re-Hypnosis:**_____

_____

**Noticeable Reaction or Abreaction:**_____

_____

_____

_____

_____

**Additional Observations:**     _____

_____

_____

_____

_____

Following is a short explanation of the chart, section by section, to point out the various implications of each response.

## Attitude of Subject

The attitude of the subject indicates how he is relating to you in the waking state, which tells you what your basic approach should be. If the subject is calm, use a maternal induction; if he is nervous, use a paternal induction; if he is fearful, project a reassuring, maternal attitude with an authoritarian induction; if he is indifferent, catch him off-guard with a subtle approach.

## Type of Induction Used

Simply list the kind of induction, indicating also whether the approach was maternal or paternal.

## Induction Timing

Your induction timing is too slow if the subject has already entered the hypnotic state before you say the words, "Deep sleep."

If he has to wait for you to catch up with him, he may lose some of his depth. If your induction timing is too fast, you may miss the subject completely and destroy some of his expectation. A perfect induction timing occurs when the subject's eyes close or roll upward at the instant the command of Deep sleep is given.

## Physical Movements During Induction

If the subject makes deliberate movements, as if he is helping you, it tells you that he is either trying to be overly helpful or he is extremely Physically suggestible and is taking everything you say literally. If his physical movements are lazy, and he shows the pulsation of approaching sleep in his movements, you have a 50/50 subject. If his physical movements are not noticeable, you have an Emotional subject.

## Subject's Suggestibility

The degree of a subject's Emotional and Physical suggestibility should be determined by a combination of the written suggestibility questionnaires, active suggestibility tests, and observation of the client while he is in the hypnotic state.

## Subject's Comfort

In a therapy situation, physical closeness means emotional closeness to a client. In some cases, emotional closeness is necessary for proper transference or for establishing a dependent relationship, just until the subject develops enough confidence to handle his own independence. Physical closeness, including touching and hugging, is common when the client is a very young child. So if a child seems to want a little physical contact, it may be anti-therapeutic not to give it. However, discretion and wisdom must always guide use of physical contact, especially with adults. Many times, for instance, an Emotionally suggestible subject will abreact to physical closeness, especially before he trusts you fully because he feels that it is an invasion of his territory. A touch on the forehead will usually indicate whether the subject is Physical or Emotional; the greater the jar from the touch, the greater the Emotional suggestibility. To ensure the subject's comfort, you should always begin with a maternal approach, which can be followed by paternalism with a Physical subject. Paternalism used first, may lack results and can be very upsetting to Emotionally suggestible clients.

## Physical Behavior While in the Hypnotic State

Look for:

1) Total relaxation (an indication that the subject is letting go).

2) Erratic abreactional movements (an indication of fear).

3) Constant movements of the body (an indication of mistrust).

## Post-Suggestion to Re-Hypnosis

The post-suggestion to re-hypnosis is fully described in the section on *The Initial Hypnotic Induction*. The primary purpose of the post-suggestion is to create rapid response to re-hypnosis, not to satisfy the operator's ego. Once a post-suggestion has been given, it must remain consistent from session to session.

## Noticeable Reaction or Abreaction

A reaction has taken place when a suggestion you have given your subject is carried out, as with a post-suggestion to re-hypnosis or a post-suggestion to reaction. For a reaction to occur, the suggestion must slip through critical area of mind and be accepted.

An abreaction simply indicates a resistance to the suggestion. If, after you repeat the suggestion one time or a number of times, the abreaction ceases, it is a good indication that you are reaching the individual, possibly even stronger than if a reaction had taken place instead. If a subject abreacts to the same suggestion throughout an entire session without the abreaction ever easing or ceasing, you should reword your suggestion.

# CHAPTER 4 – DEEPENING TECHNIQUES

## INTRODUCTION

The stereotyped concept of *hypnotic depth* is a fallacy because the established categorical guidelines (*hypnoidal, catalepsy, and somnambulism*) are limited to measuring the depth of Physically suggestible subjects only. We know for a fact that Emotionally suggestible subjects also have varying degrees of receptiveness and that the hypnoidal, cataleptic, and somnambulistic stages for Emotional subjects are much different than those for Physical subjects.

It is not how *deep* a subject is that is important, but how he responds to a suggestive idea. A person's depth is really indicated by the intensity of his receptiveness to suggestions. As a therapist, you have the distinct advantage of utilizing his most receptive state to modify the problem *if* you know how to identify it and then maintain that same condition while he is in the hypnotic state. Since the suggestibility questionnaires measure a person's potential receptiveness (the same receptiveness that created the problem), the ideal situation is to reach that particular suggestibility while working with the client to remove the problem.

Based on this new information, you will see that a more accurate title for this chapter would be *Intensifying Suggestibility* because depth is really the hypnotic influence that intensifies the receptiveness of the subject. Even the suggestion of *deep sleep* must be taken as a figure of speech, not a literal suggestion. It gives the subject the illusion that you are taking more control and that he is going more into his own being, but it is only an illusion. The words *escape* or *let go* will have an equal or better effect, as long as your pre-induction clarifies the nature of hypnosis and hypnotic depth. It is much better for the subject to think of receptiveness and intensity of response to suggestion rather than depth because so many people cannot feel physical depth. But since most people believe that hypnosis is a *deep* state, we are simply capitalizing on their expectation when we say *deep sleep*.

With this qualification established, we will continue to use the term *depth* and the three classifications of hypnoidal, catalepsy, and somnambulism, only because they have been so widely associated with hypnosis for such a long time, that a terminology change now would only confuse the issue.

## DEEPENING TECHNIQUES

At least one, and sometimes all, of the following techniques must be employed to effectively increase a subject's hypnotic depth:

1) Establishing rapport
2) Removing fear of loss of control
3) Increasing time spent in the hypnotic state
4) Successfully challenging the subject
5) Using rapid reactional hypnosis
6) Using misdirection

Building rapport, or establishing the atmosphere of the therapeutic relationship, is completely the responsibility of the therapist. A display of sound, self-confidence in the therapeutic process is essential for developing trust and positive expectation in the client's mind. However, it is particularly important not to display an attitude of egotism or dominance because so many of the myths surrounding hypnosis include ideas of dominance and control. Never make ridiculous statements, such as, "I control your mind," "You are under my power," or "You will obey my suggestions."

Also important in building rapport is professionalism in your approach to the subject. Avoid talking about yourself or other case histories. Be a good listener. If you believe you can help the subject overcome his problems, say so. If you have doubts but are willing to try, state that. Do not guarantee anything. Do not give suggestions or challenges that you are not sure will work.

Avoid discrediting other therapists or other approaches. Many times, your best results will be with those who have undergone other methods of therapy that did not work for them. Do not say that hypnotherapy is superior to other approaches, but just that it is different and may be better suited for them.

Never tell a subject that he cannot hear sounds around him, as this will only draw his attention to them when prior to such a suggestion, he may not have even noticed them. Instead, utilize distracting sounds to your advantage by suggesting that:

*These outside sounds are the sounds of everyday living. They will not distract or disturb you, but will tend to relax you.*

This further increases rapport, by giving the subject the feeling that you are directing his suggestibility.

Some clients have difficulty expressing themselves, especially in their problem area. In such cases, a non-directive approach can often encourage them to talk, without forcing or leading them. One approach would be to answer whatever the client says with a question directly related to what he just said, but asking only for clarification, until he begins to expand naturally on the subject. Another method would be to ask a series of *yes* and *no* questions, until you have enough information to identify the problem area.

Another important aspect of establishing rapport coincides with the second area of removing any fear of loss of control the client may have. Once you have the client's complete trust and have quelled any fears, depth will come naturally. The pre-induction speech is the vehicle for assuaging fears, dispelling misconceptions, and explaining suggestibility. Study the pre-induction speeches in Chapter Three carefully and never underestimate the importance of this step.

Never try to achieve depth by means of suggestions or visualizations that could represent a fear to the subject, such as, suggesting that he will have a feeling of losing control or falling, or that he will visualize going through a dark tunnel or down a well. Instead, suggest that he is walking down a staircase step by step, with his hand on a sturdy, secure, handrail, and that he is feeling very comfortable. If you see any fear reactions, hesitate between steps, thereby giving him the feeling that he can always stop.

A third technique of increasing depth is to progressively increase the amount of time you keep the subject in hypnosis. The longer the time in the state, the greater the probability of increased depth because the subject's mind has time to drift, his body can dissociate, and greater amnesia is likely to take place. A progressive time increase approach that is very effective is to time the subject at each session, starting with a fifteen-minute period the first session, and increasing it by two minutes each consecutive session, until you reach a fifty-minute period. This gives the subject the feeling of going deeper each time, and the gradual increase in time is not noticed. This is to be used only as a deepening technique, not as a standard hypnotic approach. Normally, fifteen to twenty-five minutes out of a one-hour session is a sufficient amount of time for your subject to remain in the hypnotic state.

Successfully challenging a subject, not only increases depth, but it eliminates the subject's desire to fight the hypnotic state. Instead, he escapes deeper into hypnosis. Almost any muscle or any emotion can be challenged. A rule to remember is to make sure that the subject reacts to the suggestions of tightening the muscle, or that he has built momentum for the emotional release, before you give the challenge. For example, with the eye challenge, there should be movement in the eyes, indicating that your suggestion of tightness is working, before you issue the challenge. With the emotional challenge of laughing, wait until the body shows a reaction to laughing, such as, spasmodic shivering or muscle movement, before giving the challenge.

To begin the eye challenge, tell the subject to sit back in the chair and close his eyes. Then begin with an unassailable fact that he can relate to:

*Your eyes are closed.*

and then add:

*And you feel your eyelids tightening.*

Observe the reaction of the eyelids to see if they pull down and tighten. Issue the challenge only if they do. Never guess at this. Every challenge will work, if you carefully observe the subject's reactions and act accordingly. Once you see the eyelids tighten, suggest the known again and then move into the challenge:

*Now that your eyelids are tightening, they are stuck tightly closed, and you cannot open them.*

At this point, snap your fingers or raise your voice and say:

*You may try to open them.*

Then the reversal:

*But the more you try, the tighter they become.*

And, finally, the reinforcement:

*You cannot open them.*

The suggestion that the eyes will not open becomes the dominant suggestion, and the alternative becomes the weaker suggestion. At this point, say:

*Tighter and tighter.*

Finally, suggest going deeper into hypnosis.

The arm-rigidity challenge is most effective with an Emotional subject the first time he is hypnotized; but with a Physical subject, it is equally effective the first time or at subsequent sessions.

In order to execute an arm-rigidity, hypnotize the subject through a conversion from an arm-raising test, shift him to a recliner chair, and then perform a progressive relaxation, suggesting that he go deeper. Then lift the subject's arm and extend it out fully. Support the weight of the arm by grasping the subject's elbow from the underside. Then tighten your grasp slightly and suggest that you are drawing the tensions from the subject's body and placing them into the arm. Tell the subject that you will now count backwards from five to zero, and with each count, the muscles in the arm will tighten. At two, the arm will lock, and at zero, the arm will be very rigid, just like a steel bar. Each count should be uttered more paternally, reinforcing the suggestions of muscles tightening and joints locking. At zero, snap your fingers, telling the subject that his arm is locked. With your hand in the position that it is, you will be able to feel the muscles tightening and the elbow locking before you attempt the challenge. If you do not feel tightening or locking, tell the subject to relax and go deeper. Only when you feel the elbow locking and muscles tightening, do you take the next step and issue the challenge:

> Now that your arm is tight and your elbow is locked, you cannot bend your arm. You may try, but the more you try, the tighter it becomes.

Give him a few seconds to try, and then suggest:

> When I put pressure on your pulse, your arm will relax, tensions from the body will be gone, and you will go deeper asleep.

Use of the procedure outlined above maximizes your chances of achieving an arm-rigidity, and also allows you to determine exactly when a challenge can be successfully executed.

The fifth deepening technique, reactional hypnosis, means taking the subject out of the state and then back in again rapidly many times with a post-suggestion to re-hypnosis. This causes disorientation and confusion, and is a very effective means of achieving greater depth.

The final deepening technique is misdirection. When working with Emotionally suggestible subjects, literal suggestions have very little value, so inferred or misdirective suggestions must be used. To affect the physical body of an Emotional subject for greater depth, tell him to count silently from 100 backwards to zero. Should he miscount, hesitate, or forget his count, he will go deeper, and at this time, you will touch his forehead. Watch the movement of his eyelids while his is counting. As he drifts from the count, his eyes will move from side to side. At this time, touch his forehead. Without saying anything, you have implied that he will go deeper. If you are unable to see his eyelids moving, your touch will usually throw off his count anyway, and the inference to go deeper will take effect.

Approximately 60% to 70% of the people who come into therapy are Emotionally suggestible, and properly applied inferences and misdirective techniques will give you the same result in deepening or in therapy that you would have with Physically suggestible subjects, using literal suggestions.

Misdirection is also an important adjunct to achieving greater depth with a Physically suggestible subject. In the arm-raising test, for example, suggest that one arm grows light and the other heavy, constantly misdirecting the subject's attention from one to the other, by saying:

*Your right arm and hand are growing lighter, left growing heavier; right, light; left, heavier; right, now lighter and going up.*

Continue this process, switching every so often. The suggestion of heaviness actually negates itself, since the arm cannot go any farther down than it already is; and it, therefore, causes the subject to become aware of his own resistance. The misdirection confuses the subject, who lets his guard down, allowing the power word lighter to become more dominant.

*This page intentionally left blank.*

# CHAPTER 5 – SEXUALITY

# INTRODUCTION TO EMOTIONAL AND PHYSICAL SEXUALITY

Emotional and Physical suggestibility, as applied to hypnosis, has been explained in earlier chapters. The following discussion uses the terms Emotional and Physical "Sexuality" to describe the individual's "personality" and "behavior" as it relates to their interpersonal relationships. Because this behavior is governed by the subconscious mind, it seems appropriate that the Hypnotherapist, as a subconscious behaviorist, be the expert at recognizing and utilizing this knowledge in the context of therapy.

In the current age of enlightenment, more and more people are coming to realize that the current time-honored storybook concept of "boy meets girl, boy falls in love with girl, boy marries girl" is far from reliable, let alone optimum, criteria for the establishment of a lifelong partnership. The alarming rise in our divorce rate, the tremendous increase in marriage counseling services, and the current boom for psychologists and psychiatrists, bear mute testimony to the fallacies of the old established systems. All too painfully, we have learned that love and physical beauty alone are not enough for a long-term, close liaison.

Much has been written on the subject of marital compatibility, but little effort has been give to sexual personality compatibility. It is assumed that, just because adult men and women know how to have sex and understand the mechanics of reproduction, they will automatically achieve compatibility. Nothing can be farther from the truth. Opposites in "sexual personalities" are invariably attracted to each other. This opposite quality provides the "spark," or chemistry, in a relationship. Yet, in the extreme, it also fosters emotional conflict, as two people, opposite in communication styles, priorities, and needs, misunderstand each other's motives and intent; thereby triggering insecurity. Therefore, understanding sexuality is a prerequisite to facilitating compatibility.

Because of his ego, the human being hates to think that he falls into a category; but he does. Even though his behavior may have many intricate changes and be the opposite of another person's behavior in many ways, the two categories of Emotional and Physical sexuality fit all human beings. It is important to recognize that a person will not necessarily have the same type of sexuality as he does suggestibility. An Emotionally sexual man or woman can be either Physically or Emotionally suggestible, and vice versa. We have found that suggestibility has some effect on sexuality, but the two should not be confused. Suggestibility is created by the mother; sexuality is created by the father. How sexuality is formed will be discussed later in this chapter.

## DOMINANT AND SUBDOMINANT SEXUALITY

"Sexuality" is the way in which a person behaves – not just in reference to the opposite sex or in relation to what we think of as "sexuality," e.g., love, affection, reproduction, marriage – but in all areas of life. "Sexuality" is the manifestation of sexual personality, which is simply the manner in which you, personally, order and organize, in a coherent fashion, the data you collect from your experience of the world and of other people.

Physically sexual persons project their sexual responses outwardly. They dwell on sex and desire and need physical sex often, usually as a token of acceptance or to prove that they are adequate. They cover up or repress negative emotions with this extreme sex drive. Emotional sexuals, on the other hand, feel their sexual responses inwardly. They protect the physical body by projecting emotions, such as, fear or embarrassment, to defend or repress physical feelings.

Understanding your own, as well as your client's, sexual behavior, can accurately indicate past, present, and future behavior in relationships, the sex act, and business. It can also forecast where you are going in life. A proper understanding can and will allow you and the people you counsel to change direction from a potentially disastrous pattern to a happier and more successful way of life. It can also help improve or eliminate certain sexual traits that have caused loss or hurt in a past relationship.

The Sexuality Questionnaires, later in this chapter, are designed to reveal the dominant and subdominant sexual personality and the degrees of each, which we will then go on to explain. For now, it is only necessary for you to know that you cannot pass or fail these tests. No degree of sexuality can be right or wrong. They simply exist.

When someone is 60% Physical sexual, it means that roughly 60% of the time, they will act out the characteristics of a Physical sexual. This is their dominant behavior. Roughly 40% of the time, though, they will exhibit traits of the Emotional sexual. This is their subdominant behavior. If we go back to the premise that opposites attract in behavior, we know that 60% Physical sexual/40% Emotional sexual will probably attract a 60% Emotional sexual/40% Physical sexual in a relationship. The subdominant behavior gives each of them the innate ability to understand and accommodate their partner's behavior.

This function of subdominant behavior gives background to what we will be discussing later, when we say that extremes of either behavior – Emotional or Physical – do not function well within their relationships. At 80% or above in degree of sexual personality, they do not possess enough of the opposite behavior in themselves to understand the behavior of their mate. This leads to conflict, frustration, and general unhappiness. Until the extreme sexual personality begins to understand their own and opposite behavior, they continue to repeat the same negative patterns in successive relationships.

It is also important to note here that no two people scoring the same degree of dominant sexuality are exactly the same. A simple example to which we can all relate is found in the scoring of an exam. Two students may each get a score of 80% on the exam, but answer different questions correctly to get the same resultant score. If 100% is the maximum score possible, there are many variable combinations possible that make up the individual's particular degree of sexual personality. Thus, two individuals scoring 60% Physical sexual may act out different traits of Physical sexuality, as might two 70% Emotionals act out different traits of Emotional sexuality.

So, do not anticipate that all of the personality traits listed within a given category will apply directly to you. It is imperative to your success that you rate yourself honestly, without any preconceived ideas of trying to prove anything.

## WHO ARE YOU? – MEASURING YOUR OWN SEXUAL PERSONALITY

When completing the questionnaires, please answer both of them in reference to your current or most recent significant relationship, unless the question specifically asks for data about a previous liaison. If your current relationship is still the in "honeymoon stage," then you should base ALL your answers on your experiences in one previous relationship. The honeymoon stage is usually a short period at the beginning of a relationship, but, in some cases, may continue for several years. How can you tell if you are still in the honeymoon stage? If you believe your partner is perfect, if you and your partner have never had a fight, if you still work hard to make sure your partner sees only the "good" side of you, you are probably still in the honeymoon stage. If so, then you should answer the questionnaires using the memory of some other significant, long-term relationship after it passed from the honeymoon stage into "real life."

Remember that you have no "absolute" percentages of sexual personality in your make-up. The percentages represent only how you behave, or behaved, with a particular partner. In other words, you and your partner are likely to mirror one another, percentage by percentage, on the opposite ends of the sexuality scale. A partner who behaves in an extremely Physical or extremely Emotional manner with you, will drive your own percentage of dominant sexuality upward. Similarly, you can bring your partner's escalating sexuality down into the "safe" range (i.e., 50-75%), by moderating the expression of your own sexuality.

Don't hesitate to take the test several times, relative to several different relationships, to gain extra insights into the way you behave or have the potential to behave. Just make certain that you are consistent and base each pair of questionnaires on the same relationship.

Both questionnaires contain questions that are similar to one another but are not exactly alike. Read each one carefully before selecting your answer. When completing the second questionnaire, do not check back to see how you answered similar questions on the first one.

Should any of the questions relate to an occasional behavior, do not answer "yes" to such questions because to do so will cause an inaccuracy in your final score. Read the questions *carefully and literally.* If a question asks whether you feel something or do something "more" or "more often" than your partner, then, if you feel or do that thing "the same" or "as often" as your partner, you should answer "NO." You should answer "YES," only if you feel or do it MORE or MORE OFTEN. Likewise, it the question asks whether you do or feel something "less" or "less often" than your partner, and you do or feel it "the same" or "as often" as your partner, you should answer "NO." (Reserve the "YES" answer for times when you really do or feel whatever it is less or less often than your partner does or feels this particular thing.)

If you have a cooperative partner, you may want to have him or her fill out the questionnaires, using data from your current (non-honeymoon stage) relationship. In discussing how your answers are alike or different, you may discover some very interesting things about yourselves and how you relate to each other.

## SEXUALITY QUESTIONNAIRE #1

1. In this question, we will use the term "father" to designate the male parent, step-parent, relative, or other primary role model – the male figure who had the most influence upon you and your life; and we will use the term "mother" to designate the female parent, step-parent, relative, or other primary role model – the female figure who had the most influence upon you and your life. If more than one of the answers apply, check "yes" for both. You should answer "yes," if your father exhibited one or more of the behaviors listed.

a. When you were between the ages of 9 and 14, was your father *more* possessive of you and/or *more* physically and verbally expressive of affection for you than your mother was?                                Yes   No

b. When you were between the ages of 9 and 14, were you raised by your *mother only*?                          Yes   No

c. When you were between the ages of 9 and 14, were you raised by your *father only*?                          Yes   No

2. If your partner ends a relationship that you wish to continue, do you find your thoughts drifting back to your partner and your energies turning toward restoring the relationship, to the point where you find it difficult to concentrate on other things?          Yes   No

3. Is your relationship the "Number 1" priority in your life?   Yes   No

4. Do you enjoy selecting and giving gifts to your partner?   Yes   No

5. Do you feel that you demonstrate more outward affection and love toward your partner than he/she does toward you?                                              Yes   No

6. Are you comfortable when your partner shows you attention or flatters you when others are present?        Yes   No

7. If you suspected your partner of cheating on you, would you lay more blame on the third party who led him/her astray than you would on your partner for being led astray?   Yes   No

8. Is it easier for you to express intimate feelings and attitudes than it is for your partner to do so?   Yes   No

9. Would you find it easy to accept your partner's children from a previous marriage or relationship?   Yes   No

10. Are you more jealous and/or possessive of your partner than he/she is of you?   Yes   No

11. When you and your partner are having sex, do you desire to prolong the act as long as possible or to repeat the act immediately or following a short rest?   Yes   No

12. Would you like your partner to approach you sexually more than he/she does at present?   Yes   No

13. Looking back to a previous relationship, were you ever rejected so badly that you experienced tremendous physical and/or emotional pain as a result?   Yes   No

14. In a past relationship, where you felt you had been rejected, were you capable of extreme anger, tantrums, vindictive behavior toward your partner, or violence? (Answer "Yes," if you felt capable of one or more of these behaviors.)   Yes   No

15. When you first meet a person to whom you are sexually attracted, is your attention initially drawn to the area of the body below the waist, rather than above the waist?   Yes   No

16. Are you more socially outgoing and extroverted than your partner?   Yes   No

17. When there is a problem in your relationship, do you feel that, rather than just letting things "blow over," you need to "talk it out" with your partner before you can again feel secure in the relationship?   Yes   No

18. In a relationship, do you have a need for your partner to tell you "where you stand" with him/her?  Yes  No

19. Do you want to have sex more often than your partner does?  Yes  No

20. Would you like your partner to talk about what he/she is feeling and experiencing while you are making love.  Yes  No

## SEXUALITY QUESTIONNAIRE #2

1. In this question, we will use the term "father" to designate the male parent, step-parent, relative, or other primary role model (the male figure who had the most influence on you and your life) and the term "mother" to designate the female parent, step-parent, relative, or other primary role model (the female figure who had the most influence on you and your life). If more than one of the answers apply, check "Yes" for both. You should answer "Yes," if your father exhibited one or more of the behaviors listed.

a. When you were between the ages of 9 and 14, was your father *less* possessive of you and/or *less* physically and verbally expressive of affection for you than your mother?  Yes  No

b. When you were between the ages of 9 and 14, were you raised by your *mother only*?  Yes  No

c. When you were between the ages of 9 and 14, were you raised by your *father only*?  Yes  No

2. Does your anticipation of the pleasure you will receive from sex often exceed the pleasure you actually experience from the act itself?  Yes  No

3. During sex with your partner, do you often fantasize about a different partner or sexual act, in order to become or remain sexually aroused?  Yes  No

4. Do you often find yourself wanting to hurry up and end the sex act before your partner does?  Yes  No

5. During sex with your partner, is it more of a turn-off than a turn-on, if our partner kisses you heavily?  Yes  No

6. During a single evening or session of lovemaking, after you and your partner have had sex, does he/she usually want to have sex again before you do?  Yes  No

7. Shortly after you complete the sexual act, do you feel a desire to fall asleep, move away from your partner, or to engage in some non-sexual activity (reading, watching television, taking a shower, etc.), rather than "cuddle" with your partner? (Answer "Yes," if you feel the desire, whether or not you actually do engage in the other activity.)  Yes  No

8. After the newness of a relationship wears off, do you find that your sex drive diminishes to a level where it is appreciably lower than your partner's?  Yes  No

9. Thinking back to the end of a previous relationship, did you already have a new partner in mind, or were you already involved with someone else before the relationship ended?  Yes  No

10. If your partner talks about the sex act while you are having intercourse, do you find it harder to concentrate on your sexual feelings?  Yes  No

11. Do you feel comfortable, if your partner touches, kisses, or handles you in public?  Yes  No

12. Do you find excuses not to have sex with your partner more often than your partner makes excuses not to have sex with you?  Yes  No

13. After you and your partner have resolved an argument or disagreement, does it usually take you a longer time than your partner to "forgive and forget" and get back into the mood to have sex with him/her?  Yes  No

14. Does it bother or annoy you to have to give your partner frequent reassurance and compliments?  Yes  No

15. Do you seem to need more "alone time" away from your partner than he or she needs away from you?  Yes  No

16. Instead of talking about your relationship, do you usually take the attitude that, as long as you don't complain, everything is okay?  Yes  No

17. When you and your partner are making love, does it make you uncomfortable, if your partner talks explicitly about what he or she is feeling or doing, or asks you to talk about what you are feeling or doing?  Yes  No

18. When you first meet a person to whom you are sexually attracted, is your attention initially drawn to the area of the body above the waist, rather from the waist down?  Yes  No

19. Do you think you are capable of being in love with more than one person at the same time?  Yes  No

20. Does your partner want sex more often than you do?  Yes  No

# SCORING YOUR SEXUALITY QUESTIONNAIRES

1. Give yourself five (5) points for a "Yes" answer to Question #1a, Questionnaire #1. If you answered "Yes" to #1b or #1c on Questionnaire #1, give yourself zero (0) points for those answers.

2. Add up your total number "Yes" answers on Questionnaire #1 and multiply by five (5).

3. On Questionnaire #2, give yourself five (5) points for a "Yes" answer to Question #1a. Give yourself zero (0) points for "Yes" answers on #1b and #1c.

4. Add up your total number of "Yes" answers on Questionnaire #2 and multiply the number by five.

5. Add up the number of points you scored on both Questionnaires.

6. On the Scoring Chart on the next page, look up the COMBINED scored you got on both questionnaires on the HORIZONTAL axis of the chart and circle the number.

7. Find your score on Questionnaire #1 along the VERTICAL axis of the chart and circle the number.

8. Draw a horizontal line across the page from the #1 score, then draw a vertical line down from the combined score.

9. Then number in the box where the two lines intersect representing the true adjusted percentage from Questionnaire #1, which reflects the percentage of Physical Sexuality. Subtract the number from 100% to obtain the true adjusted percentage from Questionnaire #2, representing the percentage of Emotional Sexuality.

## SCORE #1

| 0 | 5 | 10 | 15 | 20 | 25 | 30 | 35 | 40 | 45 | 50 | 55 | 60 | 65 | 70 | 75 | 80 | 85 | 90 | 95 | 100 | |
|---|---|----|----|----|----|----|----|----|----|----|----|----|----|----|----|----|----|----|----|-----|---|
| 0 | 10 | 20 | 30 | 40 | 50 | 60 | 70 | 80 | 90 | 100 | | | | | | | | | | | 50 |
| 0 | 9 | 18 | 27 | 36 | 45 | 55 | 64 | 73 | 82 | 91 | 100 | | | | | | | | | | 55 |
| 0 | 8 | 17 | 25 | 33 | 42 | 50 | 58 | 67 | 75 | 83 | 92 | 100 | | | | | | | | | 60 |
| 0 | 8 | 15 | 23 | 31 | 38 | 46 | 54 | 62 | 69 | 77 | 85 | 92 | 100 | | | | | | | | 65 |
| 0 | 7 | 14 | 21 | 29 | 36 | 43 | 50 | 57 | 64 | 71 | 79 | 86 | 93 | 100 | | | | | | | 70 |
| 0 | 7 | 13 | 20 | 27 | 33 | 40 | 47 | 53 | 60 | 67 | 73 | 80 | 87 | 93 | 100 | | | | | | 75 |
| 0 | 6 | 13 | 19 | 25 | 31 | 38 | 44 | 50 | 56 | 63 | 69 | 75 | 81 | 88 | 94 | 100 | | | | | 80 |
| 0 | 6 | 12 | 18 | 24 | 29 | 35 | 41 | 47 | 53 | 59 | 65 | 71 | 76 | 82 | 88 | 94 | 100 | | | | 85 |
| 0 | 6 | 11 | 17 | 22 | 28 | 33 | 39 | 44 | 50 | 56 | 61 | 67 | 72 | 78 | 83 | 89 | 94 | 100 | | | 90 |
| 0 | 5 | 11 | 16 | 21 | 26 | 32 | 37 | 42 | 47 | 53 | 58 | 63 | 68 | 74 | 79 | 84 | 89 | 95 | 100 | | 95 |
| 0 | 5 | 10 | 15 | 20 | 25 | 30 | 35 | 40 | 45 | 50 | 55 | 60 | 65 | 70 | 75 | 80 | 85 | 90 | 95 | 100 | 100 |
| 0 | 5 | 9 | 14 | 19 | 24 | 29 | 33 | 38 | 43 | 48 | 52 | 57 | 62 | 67 | 71 | 76 | 81 | 86 | 90 | 95 | 105 |
| 0 | 5 | 9 | 14 | 18 | 23 | 27 | 32 | 36 | 41 | 45 | 50 | 55 | 59 | 64 | 68 | 73 | 77 | 82 | 86 | 91 | 110 |
| 0 | 4 | 9 | 13 | 17 | 22 | 26 | 30 | 35 | 39 | 43 | 48 | 52 | 57 | 61 | 65 | 70 | 74 | 78 | 83 | 87 | 115 |
| 0 | 4 | 8 | 13 | 17 | 21 | 25 | 29 | 33 | 38 | 42 | 46 | 50 | 54 | 58 | 63 | 67 | 71 | 75 | 79 | 83 | 120 |
| 0 | 4 | 8 | 12 | 16 | 20 | 24 | 28 | 32 | 36 | 40 | 44 | 48 | 52 | 56 | 60 | 64 | 68 | 72 | 76 | 80 | 125 |
| 0 | 4 | 8 | 12 | 15 | 19 | 23 | 27 | 31 | 35 | 38 | 42 | 46 | 50 | 54 | 58 | 62 | 65 | 69 | 73 | 77 | 130 |
| 0 | 4 | 7 | 11 | 15 | 19 | 22 | 26 | 30 | 33 | 37 | 41 | 44 | 48 | 52 | 56 | 59 | 63 | 67 | 70 | 74 | 135 |
| 0 | 4 | 7 | 11 | 14 | 18 | 21 | 25 | 29 | 32 | 36 | 39 | 43 | 46 | 50 | 54 | 57 | 61 | 64 | 68 | 71 | 140 |
| 0 | 3 | 7 | 10 | 14 | 17 | 21 | 24 | 28 | 31 | 34 | 38 | 41 | 45 | 48 | 52 | 55 | 59 | 62 | 66 | 69 | 145 |
| 0 | 3 | 7 | 10 | 13 | 17 | 20 | 23 | 27 | 30 | 33 | 37 | 40 | 43 | 47 | 50 | 53 | 57 | 60 | 63 | 67 | 150 |
| 0 | 3 | 6 | 10 | 13 | 16 | 19 | 23 | 26 | 29 | 32 | 35 | 39 | 42 | 45 | 49 | 52 | 55 | 58 | 61 | 65 | 155 |
| 0 | 3 | 6 | 9 | 13 | 16 | 19 | 22 | 25 | 28 | 31 | 34 | 38 | 41 | 44 | 47 | 50 | 53 | 56 | 59 | 63 | 160 |
| 0 | 3 | 6 | 9 | 12 | 15 | 18 | 21 | 24 | 27 | 30 | 33 | 36 | 39 | 43 | 45 | 48 | 52 | 55 | 58 | 61 | 165 |
| 0 | 3 | 6 | 9 | 12 | 15 | 18 | 21 | 24 | 26 | 29 | 32 | 35 | 38 | 42 | 44 | 47 | 50 | 53 | 56 | 59 | 170 |
| 0 | 3 | 6 | 9 | 11 | 14 | 17 | 20 | 23 | 26 | 29 | 31 | 34 | 37 | 41 | 43 | 46 | 49 | 51 | 54 | 57 | 175 |
| 0 | 3 | 6 | 8 | 11 | 14 | 17 | 19 | 22 | 25 | 28 | 31 | 33 | 36 | 39 | 42 | 44 | 47 | 50 | 53 | 56 | 180 |
| 0 | 3 | 5 | 8 | 11 | 14 | 16 | 19 | 22 | 24 | 27 | 30 | 32 | 35 | 38 | 41 | 43 | 46 | 49 | 51 | 54 | 185 |
| 0 | 3 | 5 | 8 | 11 | 13 | 16 | 18 | 21 | 24 | 26 | 29 | 32 | 34 | 37 | 39 | 42 | 45 | 47 | 50 | 53 | 190 |
| 0 | 3 | 5 | 8 | 10 | 13 | 15 | 18 | 21 | 23 | 26 | 28 | 31 | 33 | 36 | 38 | 41 | 44 | 46 | 49 | 51 | 195 |
| 0 | 3 | 5 | 8 | 10 | 13 | 15 | 18 | 20 | 23 | 25 | 28 | 30 | 33 | 35 | 38 | 40 | 43 | 46 | 48 | 50 | 200 |

**COMBINED SCORE #1 AND #2**

# INTERPRETING YOUR SCORES

If you scored 50% or higher on Questionnaire #1, you are predominantly **PHYSICALLY SEXUAL**.

Subtract that score from 100% to find the percentage of your **EMOTIONAL SEXUAL SUBDOMINANCE**.

If you scored 50% or higher on Questionnaire #2, you are predominantly **EMOTIONALLY SEXUAL**.

Subtract that score from 100% to find the percentage of your **PHYSICAL SEXUAL SUBDOMINANCE**.

# HOW SEXUALITY IS FORMED

Generally, sexuality is determined by the father, or father figure, and is formed when the child is between the ages of 9 and 14. Boys and girls alike, who experience their fathers as more physically demonstrative than their mothers, are more likely to emerge into Physical sexual personalities. Conversely, those who feel that their mother, or mother figure, was more physically dominant and attentive than their father, are more apt to develop into Emotional sexual personalities.

When a child is raised by a single parent, there may be an aunt or uncle or teacher or friend of the family to whom the child relates to in place of the missing parent. Sexuality is then determined by the comparison of demonstrativeness between the real parent and substitute parent, as if they were both natural parents. We can see from this that sexuality, even for children separated from both natural parents, is determined by the amount of physical affection and touch received from the father figure, compared to the amount received from the mother figure. If the child received more physical attention from the father than from the mother, the child is more likely to develop into a Physical sexual. If the child received less physical attention from the father than from the mother, Emotional sexuality in the child is generally the result. Again, the important years for this comparison are the ages of 9 to 14. (For simplicity in writing, from this point in our discussion of how sexuality is formed in childhood, any reference to Father or Mother may include a substitute father or mother.

Generally, the children of an Emotional sexual father will develop Emotional sexuality, while the children of a Physical sexual father will become Physical sexuals. Let's look more closely at how this stage of development takes place.

The Physical sexual male is conspicuous in his behavior, outwardly expressing his emotions. He is physically demonstrative with people, touching them when he talks, enjoying physical contact with others. As a father, he acts out this same behavior, holding, touching, hugging, and kissing his child. He may bounce the baby on his knee, toss him gently in the air, and otherwise amuse the baby and himself through similar physical contact. This activity sets the stage for the type of sexuality – most likely, Physical – that the child will have as an adult.

As we have stated earlier, in most relationships, the man and woman will be of opposite sexuality. So, in comparison, the mother of the child as an Emotional sexual is less conspicuous in her own behavior and less physical with the child. Of course, she will pick up the baby and otherwise lovingly care for her child, yet she is more purposeful in her actions. Her intent is to respond to the baby's needs, changing diapers, feeding, bathing, or clothing her child.

As the child grows, the Physical sexual father continues to enjoy and seek out opportunities to participate in the child's life. He proudly shares his child's school, sports, and social activities. At the same time, the patterns of behavior between the child's father and his mother become obvious to the child. He notices that his Physical sexual father reaches out physically and pursues his mother's affections, soliciting verbal and physical reassurance of her love for him. She, on the other hand, seems to be quiet and shy, preferring to be pursued, rather than to pursue. The child learns that to continue to receive mother's attention and affection, he has to openly pursue her and draw her out to him. In many ways, the child thus competes with father for mother's affection and carries this method of pursuit into his own adult relationships.

With a Physical sexual father, the child becomes comfortable with physical touch and affection and acts out this behavior in relation to the mother. It does not matter whether the child is a girl or a boy. The black-and-white lesson the child learns in this scenario is to reach out for what he wants, to seek out physical touch and affection. He learns, "If you want something, go get it." Thus, the child learns Physical sexuality.

On the other hand, the child of an Emotional sexual father and Physical sexual mother sees quite a different picture during his formative years. The father's Emotional sexuality causes him to be less conspicuous in his behavior than the mother. Mother is the more physically attentive parent.

Then, as this child looks at his parents' relationship and models his father's Emotional sexual behavior, the child learns to sit back and wait to be approached. He sees his mother as the aggressor in his parents' relationship. He sees his father not reaching out or expressing emotions outwardly; he sees that his father does not particularly seem to enjoy physical touch and affection. The die is cast, and the child becomes an Emotional sexual, learning, "If you want something, wait and it will come to you."

This is the norm. Yet, at times, children will develop the opposite sexuality of their fathers. This happens because sexuality, more specifically, is a product of how the child perceives the behavior acted out by their paternal parent. This behavior, because of circumstances in the parent's relationship, socio-economic background, or because of a myriad of other reasons too numerous to list, may not always be congruent with the parent's own sexuality.

Whatever the cause, the child who learns Physical sexuality, learns to be comfortable with physical demonstration of emotions; while the child who learns Emotional sexuality becomes comfortable with introverting or not expressing emotions. Now, there is a law of human nature that motivates us to seek out and like what we know and understand and to resist or feel threatened by what we do not know and understand. It doesn't matter that something new could be good for us, we resist it simply because it is not known to us. This basic law is a strong determinant of our sexual personality. A Physical sexual understands physical demonstration of emotions and, as a child, did not know the lack of it. Thus, as adults, Physical sexuals attempting to recreate the environment of comfort they knew as children, seek physical touch and affection and are threatened by a lack of it. Emotional sexuality, on the opposite end of the scale, knows and understands a lack of outward expression of emotions and is threatened by acting out the opposite. Accordingly, sexuality is a defense against that behavior with which we are uncomfortable.

It is a primary law of nature that opposites attract; and, surely, this is nowhere more true than in the area of human sexuality. It is all part of the natural system of checks and balances that keeps the universe in balance. A male whose sexual personality rates as 70% Physical and 30% Emotional will be well adjusted in a relationship with a female who is 70% Emotional and 30% Physical. The opposite qualities of their sexuality is what provides the "spark" or chemistry between them. The more exact opposite they are in degree and type of sexuality, the greater the chemistry. In addition, they will not only be physically attracted to each other, but will also provide each other with complementary behavioral traits that each admires in the other.

The attraction of *extreme* opposites is, however, destined for disaster. If a man and a woman rate 90% or above at opposite ends of the scale, their relationship is usually one of constant emotional fireworks. They are so different in outlook and needs, that they do not satisfy the needs of the other. When conflict arises, they tend to see their partner's needs as a threat to their natural behavior and defend themselves.

The reasons for this, psychologically, are twofold: firstly, the demands of their partners usually require that they act out some of the very behavior they are trying to suppress. The Physical sexuals will demand that their Emotional partners be more affectionate; and the Emotionals will demand that the Physicals give them more space or not require sex so often. Secondly, there is another prominent law of human nature, which says that we all tend to judge others based on ourselves and our own past experience. Since extreme sexual personalities have little or no knowledge or experience of their opposite behavior, they have no basis for understanding it, much less accepting it. So, going back to our statement that sexuality is a defense mechanism, we can accurately deduce that the extremes in sexuality are too defensive and too rigid to function in a healthy relationship. Consequently, the extremes will experience the greatest degree of conflict and pain in their natural goal of achieving happiness in relationships.

Some have found a temporary solution in attracting partners of the same or somewhat lower sexuality. While this minimizes the potential for conflict, it is not a lasting solution. Same sexuality in relationships often do not provide all the ingredients necessary for a lasting union. Two Emotionals in a relationship will compete with each other, neither being able to satisfy his or her need for dominance. It takes a Physical sexual to bring the Emotional sexual out of his or her introversion, and an Emotional to allow the Physical to be more content within him or herself.

A more permanent solution to the problems that extremes will experience in relationships is to modify the behavior. In terms of sexual personality, the optimum adjustment is to be close to the 50/50 mark at the center of the "Sexual Barometer." This allows the extreme behavior to begin to soften the defense mechanisms that often exist out of ignorance or misinformation. Since we naturally fear what we do not understand, education and acceptance of the opposite behavior removes the fear and allows us to let down our guard. We can then begin to adopt some of the positive behavioral aspects of the opposite, thereby accommodating our partner's needs in the relationship. Later on, we shall devote our attention to the means by which one can effect changes in the individual sexual personality in order to achieve, or at least approach, this ideal situation.

Fortunately, through an exhaustive program of testing and consultation, we have come to understand that relatively few members of either sex are 100% Physical or 100% Emotional in their individual sexual personality ratings. In all facets of the human personality, it is rare to find a man or woman whose behavior is completely white or black. Most tend to score somewhere in the gray scale between the two extreme positions. As a person's behavior approaches the middle of the scale, which signifies a balanced behavior, he or she has a balance of needs between closeness and distance because he or she has a balance of Emotional and Physical sexuality. He or she is better equipped to attract and maintain successful personal relationships.

# THE PHYSICALLY SEXUAL FEMALE

When we say a female is Physically sexual, it does not mean that she does not feel emotions, but that she places her physical body in front of her to protect her emotions, and, therefore, requires a great deal of physical attention. A female can become Physically sexual at a very early age, if she receives a lot of physical attention from her father, and/or if she models that behavior from her father figure. Likewise, if, as an adult, a female is involved with an Emotionally sexual male and he rejects her, she will become more Physical. In all cases of deprivation or rejection, the behavior exhibited becomes exaggerated. If she is already Physical, she becomes more Physical.

In her behavior, the Physical female strives to exemplify the stereotyped image of a *perfect partner*. She is strongly influenced by how others see her, and is very eye-minded herself; so her dress and overall appearance becomes very important to her. A significant portion of her time is devoted to keeping up her appearance. She is more confident in her attractiveness than the Emotional female, and is more able to see her body as being satisfactory. The Physical female is comfortable with the roles of wife and mother and, unlike the Emotional female, feels little need to develop independence or financial autonomy. The Physical female wants to please her partner, and is deeply hurt if he criticizes the actions she has taken to please him. In every respect, the extreme Physical female attempts to embody *femininity*, and the specific considerations detailed below can all be viewed in light of this attempt.

The 90-100% Physically sexual female walks with her feet pointed outward, representing her outward acceptance of the physical. She thrives on sex and looks at men sexually. She may perform sexually once a day or as much as five times a day. When frustrated sexually, she may develop physical problems affecting the ovaries, uterus, bladder, and kidneys. She has a high vanity level and tends to exaggerate her need to prove she is feminine, and to be accepted as such. Children and family life are important to her. She has tendencies toward immaturity at times, and is usually extremely possessive and very jealous in a love affair.

If the Physical female is with a male who is withdrawn or undemonstrative, or who does not compliment her, she will feel rejected and become hurt or angry. She finds herself catering to her mate, and can be easily hurt and controlled in a relationship because of her need and desire to be accepted. Usually, she feels that she puts more energy into making a relationship work than her partner does. In fact, she becomes totally preoccupied with a relationship and devotes a tremendous amount of time and energy dwelling on thoughts of it. In the beginning, she usually looks at her partner blindly and unrealistically; and when problems or misunderstandings begin, she can never accept the fact that he is not the same person she believed him to be.

It is important to her to receive personal attention and acceptance, such as, having her hand held, her cigarette lit, doors opened for her, etc. She is overly sensitive to criticism from her partner; and when she has been hurt in a relationship, she becomes vindictive and tends to throw back at him things he said to hurt her in the past. She always hangs onto the resentment, and will bring it up over and over again years later, which, of course, creates problems in a relationship. After she calms down from an argument, however, she is quick to apologize. At that time, she becomes extremely loving and compassionate toward her partner, and may even want to make up by having sex; but her anger is quickly aroused again by rejection. If she is accepted sexually and feels sexual gratification, she interprets this as emotional acceptance. However, after an argument, her Emotionally sexual partner will find it difficult or impossible to function sexually, which, again, causes her considerable rejection.

The Physical female functions on physical feelings and, as a rule, is very intuitive. It, therefore, becomes difficult to explain any logical or rational idea or to discuss things with her when she is upset. She interprets what others say to her literally, but expresses herself in inferences, without actually recognizing the implications. Chances are that her partner is an Emotionally sexual male, who picks up inferences, but speaks literally. This conflict of understanding and expression usually shows up once an emotional trauma or argument has taken place. Prior to any emotional upheaval, both partners (especially the Physical one) have their defenses down and mutual communication is possible.

Sexually, the Physical female is capable of functioning well. However, if she reaches a point of urgency, either through rejection, sexual guilt, or feelings of inadequacy, she may focus only on clitoral sensation, and may be unable to reach orgasm unless the clitoris has constant stimulation. Since this area is difficult to stimulate during intercourse, a Physical female in this situation may begin to believe that she is inadequate sexually. Under normal conditions, however, she believes she functions perfectly. She feels tremendous arousal from stimulation in the breast area and on the clitoris. During the sex act, she requires heavy stimulation and physical handling. Unlike the Emotionally sexual female, she develops tremendous body heat during the sex act, which allows her to achieve sexual satisfaction. She will have an emotional and physical release with contraction, spasmodic shivering, body warmth, and moisture, and is capable of multiple releases. The Emotionally sexual female, on the other hand, will usually experience only climax – a lesser release or simply the end of stimulation.

Although the Physically sexual female usually experiences orgasm, she may function with climax instead, if she has some inhibitions about sex. However, climax can be converted to orgasm more rapidly with the Physical female than with the Emotional.

## THE EMOTIONALLY SEXUAL FEMALE

The Emotionally sexual female uses her emotions to defend her physical feelings. She has an inward emotional need that she feels must be satisfied; and she, therefore, covers her physical need by exhibiting the opposite behavior and withdrawing into herself.

There are certain behavioral traits common to the Emotionally sexual female. For instance, she usually has trouble expressing herself and tends to feel her emotions more deeply than she expresses them. She leads a life very different from her Physically sexual counterpart. In a relationship, she does not like to be considered a subordinate partner, but an equal partner. She tends to be deeply devoted to work and career, and may even be into women's liberation groups. Her marked need for individual identification causes her to compete in the so-called man's world. Even though she is capable of tremendous loyalty to a male boss, she is still a competitor for executive and managerial positions, and needs, both, to be accepted as an individual and to advance professionally.

She is more apt to have female companions than the Physical female (who considers other women a threat), and also openly admires other women's bodies. She looks for attractive points in other female bodies because she is never totally satisfied with her own.

Like the Emotional male, the Emotional female is more prone to participate in sports than to observe; and she prefers an element of excitement or danger in her hobbies or sports. She also dresses more conservatively than her Physical counterpart.

Most important to remember in marriage and relationship counseling is that the Emotionally sexual female has sexual cycles, meaning that she usually feels the desire for sexual stimulation once every three to seven days, and, sometimes, only once a month. When the relationship starts, she wants sex often, but as the relationship grows older, her sex drive dissipates. Immediately following the sex act, she prefers to abstain from physical touch. She cannot become aroused, if she feels overly possessed, or if arguments precede sex. Sexual stimulation begins in her mind, not in her body, so her mind must be at ease before she can enjoy sex.

The Emotionally sexual female tends to feel cold physically, especially in the hands and feet. She feels stimulation in areas that are away from the sex organs, such as; the neck, ears, abdomen, arms, legs, and feet. She may be stimulated by a light, gentle touch in the vaginal area. Many times, she will feel highly stimulated when her partner reaches orgasm, since this will divert her attention away from her own sexual feeling, and make her feel sexually adequate. Some Emotionally sexual women feel satisfied, if their partners are satisfied. The 100% Emotionally sexual female experiences little or no arousal from kissing or heavy physical stimulation, but, instead, becomes irritated by it. About 10% of the female population cannot be aroused at all by external stimulation.

Expectation of the sex act is a very important factor for the Emotionally sexual female, so planned sex should be avoided. If she feels that her partner is coming home expecting sex, and if this is part of his everyday habit, she will dread it, and will begin to think of ways to avoid sex. She may stay up so late that her partner becomes fatigued and goes to sleep. She may fake a headache or actually develop one. If she has children, she may say that they will interrupt. If she works, she may say that she is too tired. She will procrastinate and make every possible excuse not to have sex. The more she is pushed sexually, the further she will retreat into her emotional shell.

Female orgasm can be measured from 0 to 100 degrees – from a little tickle to a physical explosion and emotional release with contraction, spasmodic shivering, body warmth, moisture, and the capability of multiple releases. Usually, the high point of stimulation for the Emotionally sexual female is climax, rather than orgasm. She may have orgasm, but on the low range of the orgasmic scale; her arousal does not culminate in an explosion, but just ends. This does not mean, however, that she cannot ultimately reach orgasm to a greater degree.

In years of clinical practice, we have found that there is no such thing as a frigid female. Every female can reach orgasm to one degree or another. Being Emotionally sexual does not indicate a sexual problem; however, if a female does not understand her sexual behavior, she may believe she has a problem and, thereby, create one. If an Emotionally sexual female keeps telling herself that she is cold and frigid, or if she fears that she cannot perform, these negatives become suggestive ideas, creating a conditioned response. The mind picks up cold, frigid, and fearful, and the body reacts. Sometimes Emotionally sexual females fake orgasm and then begin to feel sexually inadequate.

For a moment, try to think about and feel what the 70-100% the Emotionally sexual female thinks and feels just before she has sexual intercourse. She has a background of sexual failure, and is, therefore, afraid of being frigid or inadequate. Her own doubts and fears make her highly suggestible. Her mind picks up the inference of failure, and the suggestions of coldness or frigidity affect her body. The subconscious mind of the Emotional female understands suggestions directly, without the filter of reason, and subconsciously constricts the blood vessels close to the skin, upon the initiation of sexual relations. Because the skin lacks circulation, it becomes cold, and any rubbing of the skin's surface, causes ticklishness or irritation. The skin then sends a signal to the brain, requesting more blood, which causes the blood to rush inward to protect the body's organs. The sympathetic nervous system is activated, adrenalin flows, the heart beats faster, and spasmodic nervousness or shivering occurs, as the organs try to force blood to the skin through the constricted blood vessels. This spasmodic nervousness or shivering creates melancholy, depression, or fear. The female tightens up and becomes sexually unresponsive. If she tries to fake sexual enjoyment, the muscles tense up and the irritation increases, compounding the problem. This is why, if sex happens spontaneously, or if she has been drinking, she may feel some sexual arousal before her mind has a chance to associate with the suggestion of being frigid, cold, and inadequate. The total reaction varies according to the degree of Emotional sexuality.

In therapy, consider the possibility that the Emotionally sexual female's own fears of performing cause many of the problems involved in sexual response. If this is the case, she should not be put in a position of performance, but, instead, a position of experimentation. In order for her body to respond to sexual stimulation, the 100% Emotionally sexual female must possess at least a small degree of Physical sexual response. To create the needed Physical sexuality, hypnotic suggestions relating to sex should be inferred, extraverbal, and indirect, in order to alter the emotional defenses of the Emotionally sexual female client.

## THE PHYSICALLY SEXUAL MALE

The Physically sexual male projects a much more *macho* attitude and appearance than the Emotional male. Usually, he is more concerned with his body and his physical appearance, than about his intellectual gifts. He is very attentive to a woman and enjoys showing her physical attention (opening doors, helping her with her coat, pulling her chair out before she sits down, etc.) and affection in public, sometimes to the point of extreme possessiveness and jealousy. He sees himself as the dominant partner in a relationship and, at the beginning of most relationships he is. However, his domination rapidly wanes, once he is rejected sexually or once his relationship is threatened.

The Physical male has a strong sex drive, and much of his energy is used in thinking about sex. He must fulfill that drive, in order to perform properly in his everyday life. He generally prefers to work with his hands, rather than in an office, and pours his energies into physical labor to vent out his sexual frustrations. When he hold back from, or is deprived of the sex act, he may become susceptible to physical ailments, especially prostate problems. Although his need for sex is always present, the circumstances of the availability may not be; and when sexual frustration is built up, it backs up into his body and creates pressure on the prostate gland. This condition is very common among Physical males, but extremely rare with Emotionally sexual males.

The strong sex drive of the Physical male enables him to have sex many times in an evening and spend entire weekends in bed, while the Emotional cannot. When the Physical male reaches orgasm, he releases only part of his semen. This is why he is able to repeat the sex act within such a short span of time. He receives greater pleasure from continual or prolonged sex than the Emotionally sexual male, who strives to end the sex act, by reaching orgasm as quickly as possible.

The Physical male receives tremendous satisfaction from sex, but, many times, he becomes controlled by an Emotionally sexual partner because of her lesser need. In the course of a relationship, he usually starts off dominant and aggressive, but becomes passive, as the relationship progresses. In extreme cases, he becomes so passive that his partner may even lose respect for him.

He has a strong drive for conquest, and, consequently, receives his greatest sexual satisfaction by assuming the top position in intercourse. All other coital positions are secondary to him. During intercourse, he often verbally expresses the different emotional and physical feelings he is experiencing. He goes to extremes to satisfy his partner, in the belief that he is doing it for her, when, in reality, he is doing it to live up to his own self-image and enhance and prolong his own sexual experience.

The Physical male feels that he is very giving in a relationship, and during marriage and relationship counseling, we usually find that it is the Physical, not the Emotional, who is trying to make it work, and who is putting more effort into the reconciliation. In general, the Physically sexual male and female usually are more capable of being faithful partners than their Emotional counterparts, as long as they receive sufficient sex to satisfy their drive. Also, marriage has a greater appeal to the Physical than to the Emotional.

Physical males are usually fond of children and, in a marriage, they want to have children of their own. They are much better able to relate to a child that their wife or girlfriend might have from a previous marriage than an Emotional male. They enjoy family life and like to share most of their social activities and hobbies with their partners. They are also very sports-minded, enjoying both participation and spectator sports. They are more prone than the Emotional male to buy season tickets for a sports event, for instance. In conversations with other men, topics of interest to them will range from sex to sports and back to sex. They enjoy the company of other men and, as a general rule, will have buddies with whom they participate in sports and social events.

The most negative aspect of extreme Physically sexual behavior is that, in a breakup following an emotional involvement, the Physical partner becomes hurt and tends to hang onto the hurt for a long period of time. He usually sees his partner very blindly during the love affair, tends to place her on a pedestal, and sees in her only what he wants to see. When a breakup takes place, he can never seem to understand that his partner was not what he thought she was, and this triggers an inner conflict between his feelings of love and the present reality of the disintegrating relationship. All of his energies and thoughts keep drifting back to her, and he is unable to concentrate on anything else. If strongly rejected, he feels actual physical discomfort or pain.

Often, the Physical male is still hurt and still in love with his lost partner many years after the end of their relationship. This may affect all areas of his functioning. Unless he understands and corrects his behavior, an extreme Physical male will usually end up in the same type of relationship over and over again because of his natural attraction to his opposite. Even if he is on guard against this, he can easily be fooled because of the Emotional sexual's pattern of behaving like a Physical in the newness of a relationship. Once the newness wears off and he recognizes his partner's Emotional behavior, it is usually too late; and the same problems start all over again.

Hypnotherapy and a complete understanding of Emotional and Physical sexuality traits can alter such extreme behavior to a sexual balance. It is easier to bring the Physical toward the 50/50 balance than it is with an extreme Emotional because it is less complicated to suppress ego sensations in the body than to bring them out, once they have been suppressed.

## THE EMOTIONALLY SEXUAL MALE

The Emotionally sexual male distributes his energies differently from the Physically sexual male. He sees a female differently and treats her differently. He has different wants and needs, and he hurts differently.

The relationship behavior of the Emotionally sexual male is very predictable. He does not like to show affection outwardly or to have to compliment a female constantly. Instead, he feels that, as long as he does not complain, she should know that everything is all right. He does not like to open doors or pull out chairs for a woman. He will restrict his wife or girlfriend from spending money on herself or the family, but he is very generous when it comes to himself and his hobbies. He always goes first-class.

His strong desire for the excitement of a new romance stimulates the Emotionally sexual male, to the point where his continual search places him in many positions to reject females. One would assume that he would be without a relationship often because of his constant search for romance and chronic rejection of his partners, but this is far from the truth. He will almost always have at least one woman on the line.

The Emotional male has a tendency to act Physical at the beginning of most relationships; and then, when the newness wears off, he returns to his original Emotional responses. The Physical, on the other hand, starts Physical and becomes more Physical. This gives the Emotional the advantage of being able to understand how the Physical functions, whereas the Physical cannot understand the Emotional because he has no way of relating to his behavior.

Once the honeymoon stage has ended, the Emotionally sexual male has a three-to-seven-day sexual cycle; he has neither the desire nor the ability to perform as often as the Physical male. When he reaches orgasm, he will release so completely, that he usually cannot perform more than once in one evening. During the sex act, he receives pleasure from stimulating his partner and satisfying her. He is affected by visual voyeurism and enjoys the role of the passive partner, preferring oral copulation or the female assuming the top position in intercourse. He is distracted and irritated by conversation or small talk during the sex act.

Sex begins mentally for the Emotional male, and he must be able to keep his mind on it, without distractions, in order to perform. He likes sex to be spontaneous and dislikes having to wine and dine a female, just to have sex. When he buys gifts for a woman, he does it in order to satisfy his guilt feelings for rejecting her; and since his partner is usually a Physically sexual female and desires sex far more often than he does, his on and off sexual cycle will cause her to experience rejection often.

The Emotionally sexual male who marries early in life will marry for different reasons than the Physically sexual male. He may marry because of an obligation or because the woman happens to be the only one he is dating at that particular time. Many times, he marries a school friend or girl he grew up with, who has pushed or chased him. But the romance disappears very quickly, and he begins to search all over again. The extreme Emotional male is usually opposed to having children and has a strong resentment toward a female becoming pregnant, whether she is his wife, mistress, or girlfriend. Because of his strong sense of obligation and guilt feelings about how he treats a woman, he is also more apt to marry her, if she does become pregnant, than the Physically sexual male would be. As a rule, however, he avoids starting a family early in life. He fears that children will tie him down and that he will waste his life with them. He seems selfishly content to have everything built around him, rather than using his energies to create a family life. Because he is not preoccupied with sex, he is rarely dominated or controlled by a female, as the Physical male can be, and his career will be less affected by the ups and downs of his relationship.

After they have been married for a while, misunderstandings and the resulting tension between the Emotional Male and his Physical wife regarding his sexual cycle, can cause the Emotionally sexual male to become sexually unresponsive to his wife. Once that happens he will begin to make excuses to avoid sex with her. He may divert his energies into his business or hobbies. His hobbies usually have an aura of danger or excitement about them. If he remains in this pattern for too long, he may then find himself seeking the company of a mistress. Of course, the Physical Sexual can be unfaithful as well, but for different reasons and in a different pattern. The Emotionally Sexual man, if he falls into this mistress syndrome, operates is a very predictable pattern. Often, when he condemns another female in the presence of his wife, it is only to keep her from thinking that anything is going on between them. Usually, the one he condemns most is his mistress. He treats his mistress differently from his wife, but feels obligated to both of them. Although it is difficult for him to express his feelings outwardly to either of them, even when he feels his emotions very strongly, usually, he will express himself more to his mistress than to his wife.

He cannot let go of his wife because he usually feels sorry for her. One of the common expressions used when he talks about his wife is, "She is a good wife [or mother], but I just don't love her, and I just can't leave her." Should he suspect that she is running around, he will accuse her or check on her, yet he would like her to make the decision to leave him. Oftentimes, if a divorce does take place, he will not marry his mistress, but will find someone else to take his wife's place. Should his mistress give him an ultimatum while he is still married, he will leave her and replace her with another. The same arrangement takes place, if he has a girlfriend he has been dating or living with for a long time. He will stay with her, but find another girl for the excitement that he feels is missing in his relationship.

To cover his tracks, The Emotional Man will develop certain patterns of times when he is supposedly playing cards, bowling, or participating in club activities. These scheduled times are usually when he is with his mistress. He seldom gets caught in his extramarital activities because he is cautious and keeps his wife in a position where she cannot check up on him. He may leave her without a car or move far enough away to make it unlikely that she will catch him. The excitement in this cloak-and-dagger operation fulfills some of his needs; but, unless he learns to understand and modify his behavior, he will live his life searching for something he may never find – and the day may arrive, when he has to face impotency and/or bankruptcy, as a result of trying to support his needs.

Whatever his degree of Emotional sexuality, he will have the basic characteristics of the 100% Emotionally sexual male outlined here; but, because of the circumstances of his relationships in the past, or because of strong family or religious ties, he may have suppressed some of them. In any case, Emotional sexuality does not diminish by itself, but, rather, grows in strength, as time passes. For his wife, it becomes a lonely existence; for his mistress, it is futile; for him, it is an unfulfilled existence and a continual search. If he learns to understand his behavior, however, he can lower his defenses and become less extreme in his behavior, making it possible to maintain a long-lasting relationship and a sense of fulfillment in his life.

# ETHNIC SEXUALITY

Ethnic sexuality is an extension of both Emotional and Physical sexuality, with added behavior traits resulting from childhood conditioning. The ethnic sexual's personality is shaped by his childhood exposure to foreign (especially Central, Eastern, and Southern European, as well as the Latin countries) cultural tradition.

To understand the ethnic sexual male and female, it is necessary to recognize the effects of the father on the family unit, since sexuality is created by the father. Unlike current American child-rearing practices, the European practices stress the primacy of the family as a whole, not the individual. In the ethnic sexual's family, there is a tremendous amount of energy devoted to maintaining family loyalty and family ties and to encouraging the offspring to follow in the father's footsteps in business, religion, morality, education, and marriage. The reasons for this exaggeration are, of course, a result of the prejudices that were imposed on these groups, when they first came to America. These prejudices kept them from opportunities in education and business and restricted their freedom to follow their ethnic beliefs. The father, being the center and the foundation of the family unit, passed these motivating insecurities on to his children because he wanted to make sure they had what he lacked. He directed his children toward family business, successful jobs, and higher education, and assured his own security in old age, by giving to his children so that they, in turn, would give back to him and take care of him later. The consistent prejudices from which the adults suffered in their struggle also caused closer relationships between father and child (more affection, more demand for respect, etc.) When a child did not obey, he was treated in such a way that he developed enormous guilt, creating in him an even greater need to be successful and to please his father.

In the beginning of a relationship, the ethnic sexual individual acts more Physical than a person of Northern European descent with otherwise comparable sexual behavior; and when a relationship is breaking up against his wishes, he feels such an overwhelming fear of loss, that he again exhibits intense

Physically sexual reactions. This aspect of ethnic behavior is most noticeable with the Emotionally sexual male and is often misleading because of his Physically sexual behavior at the beginning and end of a relationship. Once in a relationship, however, he acts very much like his non-ethnic counterpart, who takes the relationship for granted, assumes that it is the way it should be, and at times may even be abusive. The tendency of the Emotional male to be unfaithful and the Physical male to be loyal is also prevalent among ethnic sexual males.

The female, who is generally very protected in the ethnic family, reflects her upbringing, by being very dominating, outgoing, and aggressive in her relationships. Again, this is more apparent with the Emotional than with the Physical because it is not normally characteristic of the Emotional's behavior. In most other respects, the ethnic female follows the same patterns as the non-ethnic Emotional and Physical females.

In general, the behavior exaggerations exhibited by ethnic sexuals of both sexes are unusual aggressiveness, gregariousness, and a great need for personal acceptance and approval. The distinguishing characteristics of the ethnic sexual become most evident, when the security (or presumed security) of the family unit is threatened by death, divorce, desertion, or the impact of contrary cultural conditioning.

## EMOTIONAL AND PHYSICAL SEXUALITY IN TERMS OF PSYCHOANALYSIS

Because Freud's theory has been repeatedly reinterpreted, misinterpreted, and vivisected beyond recognition, a brief discussion of his basic principles should precede any explanation of the Kappasinian theory of Emotional and Physical sexuality, in terms of psychoanalysis. The length of this discussion requires that the reader temporarily view Freud's principles as axioms, in order to simplify them and in order to speak directly to the issue of sexuality.

Sexuality, in Freud's view, means much more than the sex act of the adult. His definition of sexuality is very broad, and should be understood as something that affects all aspects of human behavior. The Kappasinian theory also holds the view that sex is a primary motivator of emotional response, and not limited to direct sexual feelings. Freud believed that the sex instinct is fully expressed only in the infant. An infant expresses, experiences, and feels his sexuality in all the organs of his body. Freud's term, the infant is *polymorphous perverse*. The contentment, peace, and happiness that are often obvious in the infant's behavior, are an expression of total sexual feeling. Freud calls the infant's total sexual feeling the *Pleasure Principle*.

The basic tenet of Freudian theory is that the pleasure principle is the expression of the erotic nature of every human being. Since this erotic quality is fully expressed only in the infant, the adult is always striving to re-experience it. The subconscious mind forbids attainment of the fully erotic, in order to conform to the *Reality Principle*. The Reality Principle directs man's attention away from the polymorphous perverse goal of the Pleasure Principle and toward cultural and social organization. The imagined perfect love affair, the bliss one feels when with a lover, the poems, dramas, and works of art of modern civilization, are all products of man's effort to return to the polymorphous perverse play that is fully experienced only during infancy.

Freud views the adult sex act in terms of genital organization. This means that the total polymorphous sexual feelings of the infant become organized and localized primarily into one set of organs (the genitals, rather than throughout all organs of the body). This theory seems logical, since it explains how genital sex first appears in adolescence. Freud believes that adult sexuality exists as a result of the Pleasure Principle's antithesis, the Reality Principle. The Pleasure Principle is in conflict with the Reality Principle, and this conflict is the cause of repression. Whereas the pleasure principle represents freedom and play, the Reality Principle represents calculation and work.

Man, through a dialectical process, advances or creates his history through denial or repression of the pleasure principle. He organizes and builds a culture and becomes a social animal

(Reality Principle), as opposed to being a natural or primitive animal (Pleasure Principle). It becomes evident that Man's genital sexuality has a specific purpose: propagation of the race and the building of culture. Although propagation may appear to be natural, and thus in accord with the Pleasure Principle, it is actually in opposition to it, and is related to the Reality Principle because of its consequence of social organization. The institution of marriage, the organization of work, and the family structure, are all social, as opposed to natural, phenomena. In addition, they are not biological necessities. Biological necessity is Man's instinctual drive to reproduce and propagate his own race. It is the life force that is responsible for continuation of the species.

The hypothesis presented here is that the Freudian theory and the Kappasinian theory correlate, in that Emotional sexuality is an expressing of the Pleasure Principle and Physical sexuality is an expression of the Reality Principle.

Physical sexuality is the result of Man's lack of control of the sex drive, which, obviously, contributes, to propagation of the human race. As pointed out earlier, Freud does not view human propagation as part of the essence of the human being, but merely as a requirement of the Reality Principle. The concept of Physical sexuality is erotic and genital in character, the glorification of orgasm, the solution to all social and bodily ailments through genital organization.

The tendency of the Physically sexual individual is to express love through genital sex, and to view genital sex as an important and often-experienced part of love. Sexual rejection is the Physical's greatest fear; and any inference he takes of being rejected, will cause him to be emotionally depressed. His depression is his reaction to his fear of sexual rejection. The Physically sexual person protects his emotions, by placing his physical body (sexual feeling) in front of his emotions. His physical body acts as a radar or warning system, which allows him to hide his emotions before they can be affected. He is dependent and must feel that he possesses his partner. For him, genital sex becomes subconsciously synonymous with being loved by mother and father and being accepted. He usually marries early (thus assured of frequent genital sex), desires to have children (propagation), and is comfortable in the family environment (social organization). The central point here is that Physical sexuality has many of the same goals common to Freud's description of adult sex or genital organization, the dialectical process, whereby Man denies or represses the Pleasure Principle, in order to avoid conflict with the Reality Principle.

On the other hand, it is logical for the concept of Emotional sexuality to be correlated with the concept of polymorphous perverse infantile sex, play in the general sense, and narcissism, all of which are ways to express the Pleasure Principle. An explanation of Emotional sexuality will show how this correlation is justified.

For the Emotionally sexual individual, sex is in the mind. He is sexually stimulated first by his own imagination and visual voyeurism. The extreme Emotionally sexual personality is always searching for an emotional gratification that he is not able to receive from physical sex. He seeks a return to the repressed bliss of childhood.

The adult has localized his sex in the genitals (Physical sexuality), and he can no longer completely duplicate the polymorphous sexual feelings experienced in infancy. Although the experience of infant sexuality is recorded in the subconscious mind, it can find only partial conscious expression because of the conflict between the Pleasure Principle and the Reality Principle. Emotional sexuality is the desire to return to the experience of sex as complete satisfaction of the entire body, the polymorphous play of the infant. In the adult sex act, forepleasure is the preliminary play with all parts of the body. The Emotionally sexual tendency emphasizes generalized sex, rather than genital orgasm. Therefore, foreplay represents to the Emotional sexual a perpetuation of the pure polymorphous perverse play of infantile sexuality. This is completely experienced only in infancy, which accounts for the Kappasinian description of the Emotionally sexual person as always looking for something he cannot find. In other words, this type of person cannot find peace because the peace of childhood

(Pleasure Principle) is denied by the dictates of reality (Reality Principle) in adulthood.

Both theories contain the idea that there are two forces that constitute human emotional relationships, and that these forces are found in every person, to one degree or another. Both theories are based on the idea that these two forces are in opposition to each other, yet strive for unity. Whereas Freud's theories effectively dealt with problems of the early and middle 1900s, the Kappasinian theory of behavior has been developed with the problems of the second half of the twentieth century in mind. A person's sexual behavior is predicated on his basic human behavior, and both are affected by the changing times.

# CHAPTER 6 – FOUNDATIONS, GENERAL GUIDELINES AND TREATMENT MODALITIES

## HYPNOAMNESIA

Amnesia is a natural phenomenon of hypnosis and is apparent, at least slightly, in most clients. The degree of amnesia following a hypnotic session can range anywhere from 1% to 100%, depending on the depth and on the type of suggestibility. Subjects who enter the hypnoidal stage of hypnosis will experience 20-25% natural memory loss. They may forget incidental words and series of numbers, but power words are remembered. The subject who reaches the cataleptic stage will lose many of the suggestions prior to and following the power words. In the somnambulistic stage, even the power words can be lost and, sometimes, the post-suggestion to re-hypnosis is not remembered. The subject who awakens and remembers nothing is the exception and not the rule. The characterization of hypnotic subjects not remembering anything after awakening is an illusion propagated by the stage hypnotist.

The natural amnesia that takes place in the deeper hypnotic states is not necessarily permanent, and in a following induction or session, the memory of what took place before will frequently return to consciousness. When this happens, the subject will, many times, believe that what he remembers has just taken place, instead of having taken place in a previous session. A simple suggestion to recall what took place in the last session can bring back total memory of any hypnotic session. In addition, some clients insist on remembering everything so that they can consciously aid in overcoming bad habits or trauma, while others want to forget and just let the subconscious suggestions do the work for them.

It is sometimes necessary to induce amnesia in a subject in order to create or reinforce a conditioned response that you feel is needed to overcome a bad habit. In such cases, a high degree of amnesia can be created by using suggestions incorporating reversals. For example, the instant you awaken your client from hypnosis, tell him:

*You are already having trouble remembering what this session was all about, and it seems that the more you try, the less you remember.*

If you question your subject after giving him this suggestion, you will usually find that they have some degree of amnesia.

Amnesia can be created by suggestions from a trusted hypnotherapist, but it can also occur naturally and without suggestion, even though the client has heard everything his therapist has said. This indicates very strongly that it is the client's trust in the therapy that creates the amnesia. If trust is absent, the client will remember everything, in order to assure himself that all was proper, dignified, and appropriate. If trust and a good rapport are present, this precautionary remembering is not necessary.

## HYPNOANESTHESIA

Pain is largely a learned sensation that is created by association and identification with a suggestive idea, and it is a constant reinforcement of memories of that association or identification. Research into human physiology has rather conclusively demonstrated that only 25% of any one pain is the actual physical response of the body to trauma. The other 75% that comprises the individual's total pain experience is the emotional component – the person's fear or expectation of pain, his memories of earlier pains, his fear of permanent bodily damage or disfigurement, etc. The actual physical component of pain can almost invariably be handled, even in severe illnesses or trauma. On occasion, the physical component of pain may be minimal enough to be ignored or unnoticed. How many times have you finished an activity and only then noticed a new cut or scrape that then began to hurt? It did not hurt earlier because you were busy. It hurt when you saw it because seeing it triggered all your subconscious memories, fear, and expectations of pain – and that addition of the emotional component caused the pain. It is this 75% emotional component of pain that hypnosis handles so well.

Anesthesia is a natural phenomenon of the extremely deep states of hypnosis. Tensions tend to exaggerate pain, so when the subject is relaxed and calm in hypnosis, his tolerance toward pain rises. Consequently, the average person has fewer feelings of discomfort while in hypnosis, than he does in the waking state. This is very advantageous for medical and dental work because fears and anxieties, as well as pain, can be dissipated through hypnotic suggestion and relaxation. In addition, the gagging and salivation reflexes that so often hinder dentistry are easily controlled.

A certain amount of anesthesia is natural to the hypnotic state, and even more can be created by hypnotic suggestions. Suggestions can distract a client from thoughts of his pain (this alleviates the 75% emotional component of pain), and can even be used to transfer the pain to a less sensitive part of the body or to an area that is less threatening to the subject. Caution must be taken whenever you are removing a pain sensation, however, because pain is a signal that something is wrong, and it reminds us to take precautions to protect the injured area. Many times, it is better to reduce the pain to a tolerable level, than to remove it entirely. Before working with pain a medical referral should be sought.

Anesthesia can be created through suggestions of numbness or insensitivity, or visualization of coldness or numbness. Generally, the most effective approach to pain alleviation conditioning is first to develop an acceptable control of the body or limbs, using the arm-raising test with suggestions that:

> As your arm rises, your hand grows numb, just like the feeling you get when you have had Novocain in the dentist's office. The transfer of this numbness will anesthetize whatever area the hand touches.

This conditioning process must be repeated over and over and tied into any painful event that is anticipated in the future (an operation, dental work, or other).

Sometimes, a client's fears or expectations about upcoming pain are more paralyzing than the anticipated pain itself; and many people put off desperately needed medical or dental care for this reason. A client's last visit to the dentist, for instance, may have been emotionally traumatic. Consequently, his expectations about an upcoming dental visit involve anticipated emotional upset and trauma, and he may postpone care indefinitely for this reason. This negative expectation should be changed by means of circle therapy, whereby you desensitize the subject to the traumatic visit, then have him visualize, while in hypnosis, that the upcoming dental work is not painful, but comfortable. The association of facing the situation and feeling comfortable in it allows the mind and body to be comfortable during the actual experience.

The suggestion "You are free of pain," should be used only with a Physically suggestible subject; with Emotional subjects, you should suggest that they are *comfortable* in the situation.

## IDEOMOTOR RESPONSE

Ideomotor response is a subconscious reaction directly from the central nervous system. It occurs when the thought of a movement produces slight tension in the muscles that would be used to carry out that movement, thus actually producing the imagined movement without conscious or voluntary effort. In the arm-raising test, for example, with the suggestion that the subject's arm is lifting, up, up, higher and higher, the muscles become more tense and movement takes place, even though the subject is unaware of conscious participation.

You can utilize this automatic reaction in hypnosis (or even the waking state), by telling the subject that you are going to ask him a question or series of questions, which will go directly to his subconscious mind. From this, you expect a subconscious answer, free of any conscious interference. Explain to the client that the movement of his right index finger will indicate a negative response and the movement of his left index finger will mean a positive response. When you ask a question, the finger involved will lift automatically, giving the answer that his subconscious relates. These signals come directly through the central nervous system, without critical analysis of the conscious mind.

The same subconscious responses can be achieved with a crystal ball, a pendulum, or any weighted object tied to a string. The subject sits in a chair with his elbow on the table in a comfortable, but steady, position, with his arm at a 45-degree angle. He holds the string between his index finger and thumb. You instruct him to think Yes and concentrate on that one word only. Soon, the crystal ball will begin rotating. This particular rotational direction indicates Yes to this subject. Establish the No in a similar fashion. The meanings of different rotations differ from subject to subject, depending on whether they have right or left dominance. With all subjects, there will be slight, involuntary movements of the fingers, as the pendulum rotates. Once you have established the Yes and No responses, whether by the finger-lift or the pendulum, check them out, by asking questions to which the subject already knows the answers. You might ask such questions as: *Is your name John? Is today Monday? Are you 25 years of age?* and so on.

It is important that the subject concentrate his attention on the question itself, not on the answer; otherwise, he might influence the response by his conscious desire for one particular answer. Word all your questions so that they can be answered *Yes* or *No*. If more than one question is needed, use a narrowing-down method. If, for instance, the subject has a fear of flying, you might ask him the following series of questions:

1. *Do you have a fear of flying?*
2. *Have you had this fear for one year? Two years? Three years?*
3. *Have you had this fear long enough?*
4. *Do you want this fear?*
5. *When you become more relaxed, will this fear begin to leave you?*
6. *Can you relax with hypnosis?*

The negative conditions of the fear entered the subconscious mind at a time when the individual experience created a highly negative suggestible state. Now, by creating a highly positive suggestible state through hypnosis, the fear can be neutralized by implanting positive ideas, even while you are still engaged in ideomotor questioning (Questions 5 and 6 begin this process). The subconscious mind has received impressions since the day we were born and, possibly, ever since we were in the womb. It has recorded and stored the most minute details of feelings and events that our conscious mind has long-since forgotten. In theory, the mind resembles a computer. During ideomotor response, it draws on information that it has accumulated, regarding all the conditions of the past that relate to the question being asked, and then it produces an answer. It functions much like a mathematician, who takes a project, adds all the known factors, computes them, and comes up with an answer.

When ideas and images that the mind holds are stimulated and organized by a question, impulses travel through the nervous system and can be seen as physical reactions. Most often, these responses can be observed only through electrical devices, such as the polygraph. Through the ideomotor response technique, however, these responses from the subconscious mind via the nervous system can be detected with a minimum of effort, since the subconscious mind, not only accumulates and holds memories of all the events of our lives, but also controls bodily movements of which we are not even aware.

One of the greatest advantages of the use of ideomotor response is to identify any negative traits, conditions, ideas, fears, or causes of behavior that might be hindering the client, but which might be consciously inaccessible. The ideomotor questioning technique can be used with questions on any topic, and you can achieve results with it, as long as the answer is in the subject's mind. Ideomotor questioning cannot tell you what is in someone else's mind.

The mind is remarkably accurate in its answers because of the accumulation of the countless bits of information that it has stored throughout the subject's lifetime. Also, it is interesting to note that, if this experiment is properly done, even if the subject feels that the answer should be *No*, the subconscious mind will relate *Yes*, indicating true subconscious response. This also substantiates the theory that most of our emotional problems are created by conflicts between the conscious and subconscious minds. It must be noted, however, that the answers obtained through ideomotor response should not be construed as absolute truths. They should be instead viewed as the client's subconscious beliefs on the subject. A client, for example, who provides information through ideomotor response, that the cause of his or her problem is rooted in a childhood trauma, provides the hypnotherapist only the confirmation that the client's subconscious believes that to be true, not that it is an absolute fact.

# BIOFEEDBACK (GSR)

There are four different areas in which biofeedback can be very helpful, when used in conjunction with hypnosis. They are:

1. *Testing Suggestibility*
2. *Testing for Hypersuggestibility*
3. *Identifying Traumas*
4. *Aiding in Self-Hypnosis*

The biofeedback instrument that the Hypnosis Motivation Institute has found to be the most effective is the GSR meter – a small, battery-powered, solid state unit, which measures galvanic skin response (GSR), and which is acutely sensitive to emotional or physical stress or excitement. It has two electrodes, which are attached firmly around two fingers of the same hand, and the meter has settings, ranging from one to nine. A larger unit, called a biosonometer, also has a meter for gauging feedback visually so that the speaker tone may be switched off and the visual feedback meter used alone.

The threshold tone of the GSR meter determines the body's state of relaxation, and the tone changes in pitch, in relation to the changes in skin resistance. The signal change indicates the activity of the sympathetic branch of the autonomic nervous system, and this feedback allows you to observe your subject's reaction (or your own) to emotional stimuli. If you turn the knob of the GSR meter slightly to the right, you will hear a rhythmic, ticking beat, and as you continue to turn it, it will become a steady tone. The tone will vary in pitch. A higher pitch indicates activity or stress; a lower pitch indicates relaxation. There is usually a one- to three-second delay between the time the stimulus occurs and the time the tone rises in response.

The setting that produces a normal tone will vary with each subject. There are no absolutes. Approximations, to be used only as guidelines from which to begin, are as follows: 1.5 to 1.9 for the physical subject, 2.5 and up for the emotional subject, and 2.0 to 2.2 for the balanced subject.

The GSR meter clearly distinguishes between Emotional and Physical suggestibility, and can be used as an aid to testing suggestibility. The Emotionally suggestible subject, who enters hypnosis through expectation and inference, will rapidly bring the tone down to a very low ticking, or even to no sound at all, as he becomes more suggestible or receptive in the hypnotic state; and he will be able to maintain this low ticking during the entire induction. The Physical subject, on the other hand, enters hypnosis as a result of anxiety, fear, or any physical feeling that stimulates excitation; so the tone will increase at first, indicating activity, and then decrease or normalize, as relaxation takes over.

Once the induction has ended and the subject is in the hypnotic state, the tendency is for the GSR resistance to go down for, both, the Physical and the Emotional subject. For the Emotional, it may drop all the way to zero; with the Physical, it may go down to one or two. It is relative to the level the meter registered during the induction.

Emotional and Physical subjects differ in the awakening procedure, as well. When you awaken the Emotional subject, the tone generally begins to rise and then returns to normal. This indicates how long it takes the subject to come out of the hypnotic state. The normal awakening time is one to three minutes. As you begin to awaken the Physically suggestible subject, the meter may drop considerably; but as he awakens, it will go very high and then level off. If the tone has not returned to normal after three minutes, the subject may be trying to escape back into hypnosis, and you must use a jarring method to awaken him completely.

The biofeedback approach works especially well during the first session; but, once a subject is accustomed to using it as a gauge to enter hypnosis, the meter will not react as strongly in either direction. The hypnotist should always explain the results of the responses to the client, after he has come out of the hypnosis, in order to further reinforce its effect.

Another important way that biofeedback can aid the hypnotist is by revealing Hypersuggestibility in a client. A hypersuggestible individual is in a waking trance-state and can easily be affected by negative influences in his environment. Both Emotional and Physical subjects, who are in this state, will respond to the GSR meter by very rapidly lowering the tone and maintaining it without change. If this occurs, follow the Dehypnotization process (outlined in Chapter Seven) until the meter gives a normal tone for that person.

Another use of the biofeedback is to help identify traumas or traumatic experiences. To do this, set the gauge at the level that gives a fairly rhythmic beeping – about two beeps per second. While the subject is in a conscious state, tell him that you are going to ask him a series of questions dealing with the symptoms he is reflecting. Instruct him not to think of the answer, but to concentrate on the question itself. When you find the cause with either an Emotional or Physical subject, the emotional response will be recorded by the tone of the meter. The more severe the trauma, the greater the rise in tone. This will continue until the individual's trauma has been dissipated. When the alternatives to the cause are given consciously, the Emotional subject is more likely to bring the GSR reading down than the Physical, but it will increase measurably in both cases.

Once you have located the cause, place the subject in a light state of hypnosis and give him positive alternative suggestions, until the gauge ceases to raise the level of the meter. This indicates that the mind has accepted the alternative and that the cause is diminishing in power. An alternative to this approach would be to give positive, literal suggestions, directed at removing the cause.

The biofeedback meter is also an effective aid to self-hypnosis. In essence, it becomes a tool for creating the suggestible state of total relaxation, where self-awareness and self-control begin to increase, causing a greater degree of suggestibility to oneself. As an individual achieves relaxation in self-hypnosis, the tone will decrease and eventually cease, in proportion to the degree of relaxation. If he practices bringing the meter down at all different ranges, he will develop greater control of his body and, through the Law of Association, greater control of his emotions. He should practice obtaining and sustaining this control in self-hypnosis, by giving himself suggestions of calmness, relaxation, and self-confidence, while using the GSR meter to measure his progress.

The main difference between the smaller GSR meter and the larger biosonometer is that the smaller one is much more sensitive. Even a change in the operator's tone of voice may alter its tone. It is most valuable as a gauge for determining the subject's suggestibility, as he is entering the hypnotic state. The larger unit is used mostly in the conscious state, to seek out traumatic events in the subject's life. Once you become proficient with the smaller unit, you should switch over to the larger one exclusively because it is less sensitive and, thus, easier to monitor.

## BODY SYNDROMES

The theory of *body syndromes* is based on the principle that, whenever an emotional trauma is present, a corresponding physical reaction will take place. These physical reactions, called *body syndromes*, will, in turn, reflect the cause of the emotional problem, according to the area or areas of the body that become affected by pain, pressure, or tension.

There are many examples of how the body reacts to the mind without any logic or reason. One example is the reaction to the expectation of fear. The mere anticipation of a feared object or event can cause bodily changes, such as increased respiration and heartbeat, variance in body temperature, activation of the adrenal glands, and increased production of insulin by the pancreas. All of these physical changes originate from thoughts and their effects on the brain. These thoughts initiate very primitive physiological responses in certain parts of the body, which are similar to those that take place during a fight or flight reaction. These physiological responses are a carry-over from the time when man reacted to outside stimuli with his body, instead of his mind.

The modern verbal extension of the body syndromes is expressed in *organic language*. Organic language describes an emotional thought that causes a physical reaction in a certain area of the body. These expressions usually take the form of little clichés relating to the body. For example:

    a. *All this responsibility gives me a pain in the neck.*
    b. *I can't stomach that.*
    c. *I am sick and tired of that.*
    d. *He is carrying all the responsibility on his shoulders.*
    e. *He is blinded by passion.*
    f. *This work is killing me.*
    g. *I have a blinding headache.*
    h. *I am so confused, I can't see straight.*
    i. *I'm losing my mind from worry.*

Along with the development and evolution of language, we have constantly stimulated the body syndromes through organic language so that, at times, thought, language, and action become one.

There are five major body syndromes. Each will be described according to its physiological and its psychological symptoms.

## 1. Crying Syndrome

This first and major syndrome involves the area of the body from the solar plexus upward, covering the chest, head, and back of the neck.

The cause of the crying syndrome is the inability to make a decision, either because it is predicated on someone else's action or because of an inability to make decisions, due to past conditioning.

Headaches are the most common characteristic of the crying syndrome. Because of frustrations from indecision, the brain signals the muscles in the scalp to tighten, causing pain. Sometimes, the tightening becomes so severe that it constricts the head, resulting in migraine headaches.

Some of the other easily recognizable symptoms of the crying syndrome are: crystallization of the eyes or relaxation of tear ducts, causing the eyes to water; sinus congestion; constriction of throat muscles; gastric pressures in the chest area; tightening of muscles in the back of the neck; canker sores in the mouth; tightening of jaw muscles or grinding of teeth.

Each one of these physical reactions can be associated with an emotional or mental cause. For instance, the head pressures represent inability to make the decision; watering eyes and sinus congestion symbolize not wanting to see the situation that is causing the indecision; constriction in the throat, tightening of jaw muscles, or grinding of teeth, result from not wanting to express anything about the area of indecisiveness.·

If improperly handled or not handled at all, indecisiveness moves into frustration, and from there, to melancholy, depression, and, finally, futility. Chronic indecisiveness can be classified as a major problem in today's fast-moving society, especially among individuals aged fifteen to thirty-five.

## 2. Responsibility Syndrome

The bodily areas affected by this syndrome are the shoulders, the upper back, and the upper spinal area. The psychological causes are too much responsibility, fear of the weight or responsibility; or neglecting; not accepting or not facing responsibility.

The physiological reaction of the responsibility syndrome is tightening of the back and shoulder muscles. In some instances, if excessive or rapid movement or lifting is attempted when these tensions are present, physical damage can be done to the back.

## 3. Sexual Frustration or Guilt Syndrome

The areas of body affected are the stomach, groin, and lower back. The psychological causes can be sexual frustration, religion-linked sexual guilt, guilt about infidelity, feelings of sexual inadequacy, and so forth.

The physical symptoms can be stomach cramps, constipation, acid stomach, excessive menstrual cramps or bleeding (or no bleeding at all), vaginal or bladder infections, prostate or testicle pressure and pain, and kidney problems.

## 4. Fight or Reaching Syndrome

The areas affected are the arms, hands, and fingers. The psychological symptoms involve the need to express with concomitant denial or suppression of that need; the inability to reach for something one desires because of a lack of feelings of self-worth; and a feeling of deep rejection, as a result of reaching for unattainable goals.

The physiological effects are warts or little blisters on the hands or fingers, tightening of the joints and muscles in the hands, or extremely hot or cold hands. Arthritis and rheumatism are related problems.

## 5. Flight Syndrome

This syndrome affects the area from the thighs to the feet. It indicates a need to run or escape (emotionally or physically) from a particular situation or involvement. The psychological causes are a fear of facing certain situations because they may be painful, boredom, fear of disaster, and fear of success.

The physiological symptoms are blistering between the toes or on the bottom of the feet, cold feet because of poor circulation, and leg pains.

At any given time, a person may be affected by one or more of the syndromes described above. For example, a headache and tight back muscles, in combination, indicate an inability to make decisions about responsibility. Tension in the back muscles and pain in the legs denote that responsibility is causing a person to want to escape from a situation that he cannot actually leave. In my opinion, most physical ailments are caused by body syndromes that remain too long without proper treatment.

Observation of your client's physiological reactions, reflected in body syndromes, will usually reveal the basic psychological cause. By consciously explaining the syndromes to your client, you can, in most cases, eliminate or ease the physiological distress. By subconsciously suggesting alternatives to the psychological cause, you can generally eliminate both distress and cause.

An understanding of the body syndromes provides you with a diagnostic approach that can be used in conjunction with all types of therapy. In addition, it helps you to recognize that the suggestive ideas that you give your client will affect, not only his mind, but also his body.

## SYMPTOMATIC APPROACH

The *symptomatic approach* simply means working directly with the symptoms of a particular problem, and not with the primary or secondary causes. It is the first and easiest approach to take in therapy. No harm to the subject can possibly come from it because, if the symptom should grow strong during the therapy, it will then become apparent to the therapist that the symptom is a mask or a hysterical conversion employed by the client, in an effort to avoid facing the cause. If this is the case, the cause must be searched out. Only a small number of cases, however, require an identification of the cause because the majority of problems can be alleviated symptomatically. In fact, many symptoms have been known to disappear, simply because of imagination, medical placebos, or a change of environment.

The most basic symptomatic approach involves *systematic desensitization*. With this method, you simply place the client in hypnosis and suggest that the symptom distressing him will soon disappear. Then have him imagine feeling comfortable in a given situation that usually causes his symptomatic discomfort. Many times, people will have anticipatory dread of an event, and this dread will cause misery during the event. The discomfort experienced will increase the anticipatory dread, and a vicious cycle, operating on the Law of Association, begins.

In therapy, this is corrected by having the client imagine an association of the negative situation with feelings of comfort and ease. Since feelings of comfort and discomfort cannot coexist, the negative stimulus will lose its potency, and the symptomatic discomfort will disappear.

# PRIMARY AND SECONDARY CAUSES

Occasionally, a client's symptoms expand or worsen when the symptomatic approach is used. In such cases, the primary and secondary causes must be sought. The *secondary cause* is the recent event or condition that triggered the present disturbing symptoms. The *primary cause* is the initial event that made the individual susceptible to the disturbing symptoms. It is important to remember that the primary cause may have occurred many years before the outbreak of the unwanted symptoms – perhaps even in infancy. This means that it may be inaccessible in conscious therapy, and will have to be searched out by way of dream therapy or age regression. Careful observation of the secondary cause will usually give clues as to what the primary cause is, or where to search for it in age regression.

The two examples below will clarify what is meant by primary and secondary causes. They indicate appropriate treatment approaches.

*Example #1:*  Symptom:  Fear of flying.
 Secondary Cause:  Recent air flight with great deal of turbulence.
 Primary Cause:  Earthquake experience at the age of four.

The subject is not actually afraid of flying, but has associated the recent turbulent flight with the horrifying loss of control created by the primary cause. The client associates the feelings of loss of control with flying, and, therefore, believes that he is afraid of flying. He does not recognize his fear of loss of control. In a therapeutic situation such as this, the symptomatic approach is contraindicated because the symptomatic suggestions do not attack the true problem. In fact, such suggestions may create an additional fear, since the client is being told that he has a fear of which he has not been previously aware. The proper approach is to use circle therapy to desensitize the client to the fear of loss of control, arising from the primary cause.

*Example #2*   Symptom:            Fear of crowds/crowded places
            Secondary Cause:  Physical sickness, invariably
                                experienced in crowds.
            Primary Cause:      A frightening hypoglycemic
                                attack experienced in a crowded
                                place earlier in life.

In this therapeutic situation, the symptomatic approach is, again, contraindicated. Instead, the initial association between sickness and crowds should be uncovered. Then, the link between primary and secondary causes should be demonstrated. By avoiding crowds, the client is trying to keep from being sick and out of control, a condition which he associates with crowds because of the timing of the first attack. Once this is realized, it may be unnecessary even to use circle therapy to defuse the primary cause of this unwanted and unnecessary symptom.

Whether you are beginning a therapy or preparing a written case history, always record the primary and secondary causes (if known), even if you do not intend to work directly with them. It is valuable to be aware of the cause because this can sometimes help you in a symptomatic approach, and will always help you to better understand your client.

## CIRCLE THERAPY

Circle therapy is the process of having a client repeatedly confront his problem and experience his anxiety in controlled amounts while remaining in the relaxed hypnotic state. Since anxiety and relaxation are incompatible, the anxiety will gradually disappear.

Before placing your subject in the hypnotic state, tell him that, in a moment, he will begin to enter a scene in his mind that represents his particular problem or state of mind. Assuming for example, that he has a fear of dark rooms, you would take him into the hypnotic state and give him a variety of positive suggestions to eliminate this fear, always indicating verbally, as well as non-verbally, that, after the session is over, the fear will be completely eliminated. Then take your client into the circle, having him imagine and feel, not only the situation of the dark room, but the fears that accompany it. When he begins to abreact to the situation, take him out of this unpleasant state, by suggesting that it is over now and that he is feeling calm and relaxed. Do not take him out of hypnosis. After a few moments, repeat the entire process, telling him:

> *You will find this time that, as we begin to approach the fear of the dark room, it becomes very difficult for you to feel the fear because you have neutralized it. And, of course, the more you try to feel it, the more amused you become by the fact that it no longer affects you.*

You will notice that with each repetition, he will have less and less fear and that the smiling, which indicates the release of the fear, will begin.

After you repeat this circle therapy two, three, or four times, depending on the severity of the problem, replace your subject's fear with very positive thoughts, ideas, and logical explanations of the situation. Always add that, each time he tries to feel the fear, he will find he becomes amused by the fact that he cannot feel it. This amused self-satisfaction becomes a replacement for the earlier anxiety caused by the problem situation.

When the subject faces his fear in the controlled situation of the hypnotic state, it:

1. Weakens the symptom, and then allows the client to face it again, once the abreaction has ceased.

2. Allows the subject to face the cause without experiencing the symptom.

3. Increases the subject's ability to adapt. This ability may spill over to other situations.

4. Can relieve the fear of loss of control and the dread that the fear will someday control the subject completely.

5. Helps remove the fear of facing the trauma alone.

6. Allows for a positive behavior to be substituted for a negative one.

7. Causes venting through dreams.

8. Allows positive secondary suggestions to enter the mind without being critically analyzed.

9. Allows a healing amnesia to be created more easily because the subject is anxious to escape and to forget the trauma.

10. Is a form of *systematic desensitization*.

# CIRCLE THERAPY ILLUSTRATION

1. Illustration of how a trauma is triggered in the conscious state by the expectation of the trauma taking place.

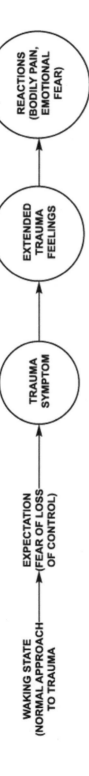

2. Illustration of how to control and diminish a trauma by means of Circle Therapy.

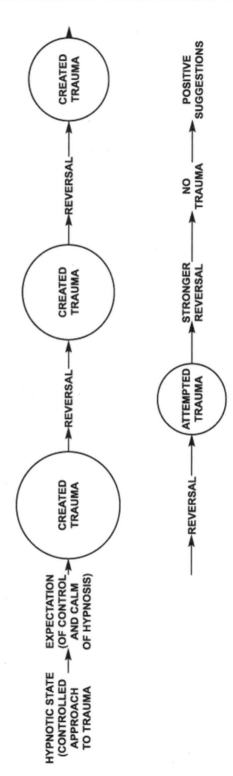

Circle therapy should be used any time the direct symptomatic approach to therapy does not work. An example of symptomatic suggestions for this same problem would be:

*You will no longer feel, experience, or remember this fear. The memory of it fades very quickly. It is in the past now.*

Circle therapy brings about spontaneous regression to a specific problem, but because the problem is known is does not have the dangers of age regression.

## AGE REGRESSION

*Age regression* has for decades been the modality of choice for hypnotists. Because of this prevalence, many people associate hypnotherapy with age regression, thinking of them as one and the same. The fact of the matter is that age regression is the most problematic and dangerous techniques in the field. The reasons are two fold.

First is the premise that hypnosis works like a truth serum or a search engine into the subject's personal history. Unfortunately, this could not be further from the truth. One of the properties of the hypnotic experience is the subject's increased capacity for confabulation.

The ability to imagine and experience things that are not real makes hypnosis a wonderful tool for change and at the same time a terrible truth serum or historic fact finder. To make matters worse, once a subject emotionally experiences some past experience, whether it is factual or not, or whether his experience is exaggerated or distorted or accurate, this new version now becomes his reality and version of history.

It is because of this use of hypnotic regression that hypnotists and therapists in general created a syndrome known as "false memory syndrome." This syndrome has resulted in multi-million dollar liability awards as client's successfully sued therapists who used age regression hypnosis and claimed emotional trauma to them and their loved ones. It was this same issue that caused

California to ban hypnosis obtained testimony as admissible evidence in a court of law.

In addition to false memory syndrome, there is another problem with the premise of using age regression hypnosis to uncover repressed memories of past traumatic events. If these traumas are truly not known or remembered by the subject due to the defense mechanism of repression, then they are most likely fairly traumatic and significant experiences that have been repressed in order to protect the individual from that which he cannot handle. True "repression" is not a common experience. It is typically only employed as a defense mechanism in cases of either extreme trauma or fragile personalities. In either case, putting a person in a highly suggestible state and then flooding her with a repressed traumatic experience certainly presents a questionably risky therapeutic technique.

The only time that hypnotic age regression can be a justified therapeutic technique is when the historic traumatic event is known to the client, and you go back to desensitize the experience and its resulting impact. Never should age regression be used as a search tool to "find cause." Other methods presented in this text, like dream therapy, corrective therapy and other diagnostic tools would be recommended instead.

## VISUALIZATION

Some of the misconceptions about visualization are that imagination and visualization are identical, that only a highly imaginative person can visualize, and that hallucination and visualization are the same.

Since hypnotized subjects are frequently asked to visualize and/or imagine, it is important to clarify just what is meant by these two activities. For our purposes, visualization is the ability to actually see an object or scene when the eyes are shut. Some people are able to see motionless objects or static scenes only. Others may see the equivalent of color movies. Imagination is the ability to think of objects or scenes and to remain fixed on this thought for an appreciable period of time.

Everyone can imagine to one degree or another. Not everyone can visualize. A person's ability or inability to visualize tells us about his learning process – whether he is ear-minded or eye-minded. If he is eye-minded, he tends to learn what he sees, and later see what he has learned. Visualization, then, is a normal outgrowth of eye-mindedness. An ear-minded person learns best by listening and hearing. Visualization would be a distraction to his inner voice and would not be a natural outgrowth of his optimum learning pattern. Thus, the ear-minded person will generally not visualize.

Both, ear-minded and eye-minded people can imagine an object or scene, and both do equally well in hypnosis. The ability to visualize appears to have no correlation with depth in hypnosis or with Physical or Emotional suggestibility. In the hypnotherapeutic setting, it is important to determine prior to the first induction whether the client can visualize. If he cannot, simply tell him to *imagine* whatever picture or scene is appropriate to the therapy. Many hypnotists will suggest that a subject visualize without first finding out if he is capable of it. If a client cannot visualize, a command to do so will restrict his hypnotic suggestibility.

Visualization and hallucination are not the same. Visualization in hypnosis is a controlled behavior, and the client will not believe that the visualized scene or event is currently happening or is factually true at this point in time. (It may, of course, be a scene that he hopes will be true in the future.) *Hallucination* is generally an uncontrolled behavior, with the victim either unaware of the delusion of his inner visions or unable to control them.

Visualization can be developed through practice of what is called *aftervision*. This involves staring at an object or a picture for thirty to sixty seconds, then closing the eyes and seeing it on the back of the eyelids, or opening the eyes and seeing the negative of the article on a blank wall. A series of practice sessions in the aftervision can create better visualization, if it is desired. However, visualization is in no way essential for hypnosis or for any other type of therapy.

# SUGGESTIVE IMAGERY

It is essential that you, as a therapist, have an understanding of mind symbols and how to uncover them in therapy. They are especially important as an adjunct to dream interpretation and self-hypnosis, as well as in the structuring of inferred suggestions. Do not confuse imagery with visualization. Visualization is the result of deliberately attempting to see something in the mind's eye; imagery occurs as a spontaneous reaction to verbal or extraverbal input, and does not always involve a visual image. Images or symbols in the mind vary with each individual and are based on his reactions to his unique life experiences and on his type of suggestibility. This is why two people from the same family, raised in the same traditions, and educated by the same teachers will generate different symbols from the words they have learned. When these images are recognized by the therapist, they can be used very effectively as suggestive ideas for that individual.

In order to recognize an individual's unique images, you must first understand how they originate. Every thought a person has produces an image of what that thought represents to him. For example, if you think of the word *mother*, an image comes into your mind. Even if you try to concentrate on the word without the image, the image cannot help but come to mind, nor can the thought be separated from the image. Consequently, a cause and effect reaction begins. The thought is the *cause*, the image is the *effect*. The image can immediately create another thought, which produces another image, and so forth. This continual bombardment of thought and image results in either a physiological or a psychological reaction or feeling. If there is an emotional reaction of sorrow or of happiness, the body will respond by being upset and depressed, or elated and vigorous. This happens most often without the person realizing why. If the negative emotion is triggered often enough, the individual will develop a habit of feeling bad physically, as a result of feeling bad emotionally, and the physical problems will result in more emotional problems, and vice versa. It becomes a vicious cycle that cannot be stopped without recognizing and altering its source.

Symbols have been an intricate part of Man's expression since the beginning of time, from hieroglyphics to the classical artists and present-day artists, and even to samples of strokes of handwriting. Imagery is the pure interpretation of primitive thought that still influences the modern mind.

The more we acquire and learn, the more complicated and intermingled our symbols become. Pure psychosis can simply mean that what a person sees and hears consciously is in total conflict with his subconscious images. This dichotomy is exaggerated to the point where all the images that he has accumulated in this life begin to dominate his way of relating, causing him to deny the reality of his conscious perceptions.

The use of imagery in therapy is not new. It has been explored in almost all modes of therapy, notably in *word association* exercises (where it is actually the image associated with the word and not the word itself that affects the physical or emotional response), most methods reach the subconscious only through chance association, whereas hypnotherapy deliberately delves into the subconscious mind.

A hypnotic suggestion cannot work without imagery. When you, as a therapist, are talking to a subject, what you are saying goes from a thought, to an image, to an emotional and physical reaction. As such, it becomes a very strong suggestive idea. Many times while talking to a client, you will say something, and immediately his eyes glaze, his face becomes drawn, and he looks as if he is going to break down emotionally. This is because, as he was listening to you, you caused him to think about something, and an image associated with that thought formed in his mind, triggering an emotional and physical response. It usually happens so rapidly that all the subject is aware of are the emotional and physical feelings and the original thought. Symbols always pass very quickly, especially if there is an over-abundance of message units going into the brain, so you must make the subject aware of the symbol, by going back over what triggered him, and having him verbalize his thoughts and reactions. Once his thoughts are expressed, the imagery becomes less important and will not feed back another thought into his mind. The feeling that would normally be created is then suppressed, and the imagery passes, preventing any physiological or psychological feeling from being associated with the thought.

The emotional response described above can also happen when you are searching for reasons why a client is having a particular reaction, and you suddenly hit upon the cause. At that time, the image flashes into his mind, his eyes will crystallize, and the symptom may dissipate instantly. The same results can be obtained by identifying the body syndrome area, where the symptom is reflected, and then going over every possibility of cause, until you see the client's eyes glaze. Even though the problem might be associated with any one of the syndrome areas, eye crystallization will still take place when the cause is recognized because, at that precise moment, the client is making a decision (to let go of the problem), and the decision-making is reflected in the crying syndrome area. Once a subject becomes aware of his own suggestive imagery, he can utilize it in self-hypnosis, by using only positive symbols that give him clear images and good emotional and physical feelings. In self-hypnosis, he would not verbalize the images, but would put them into his mind as thought imagery. He must be aware of the image and the feeling he has from it, and then never repeat it out loud, until the process becomes so deep in his mind that, by repeating it, he cannot remove it.

In trying to understand symbols, it helps to understand how an inference works, as well. If you suggest to a subject that he will gain more confidence in a certain situation, or if you desensitize the area where he lacks confidence, you are using literal suggestions. To attack the lack of confidence by inference, you must discover how lack of confidence makes the client feel, and then identify the imagery that the lack represents. If lacking confidence, for example, makes him feel inadequate or embarrassed, suggest that he will feel adequate and comfortable in a given situation. This will imply that he has confidence. A person cannot lack confidence without an image of it or without emotional and physical responses to it. If you remove the images representing the lack of confidence, the subject will notice their absence and will realize (by inference) that he is more confident.

The *corrective therapy* approach is a good exercise for your clients to practice, in order to discover their symbols and find out what these symbols mean to them.

## CORRECTIVE THERAPY

*Corrective therapy* is an approach, whereby a sentence produced by the conscious mind reveals the subconscious symbols of the mind. Each person has his own unique mind symbols, and a determination of these symbols will give you valuable insight on how to structure suggestions.

The mechanics of corrective therapy consist of having the client write down a sentence that states his problem, and then having him list a series of four or five synonyms in a column under each word. The Physically suggestible individual should write a series of synonyms for the word in the original sentence; the Emotional should write a synonym for the first word, then one for the second word, and so forth.

The reason for the difference in approach is that the Physically suggestible individual will express himself very literally in the first sentence, as well as in his listing of synonyms. Since he also accepts literal suggestions, the corrective therapy will be of most value to him in this form. The symbols for an Emotionally suggestible subject, however, are more complex because of the nuances of their inferred meanings. The more indirect approach to corrective therapy is effective for the Emotional subject because it breaks the sentence and the words of the sentence down into abstracts, in order to expose their true inferred meaning to that particular individual.

An example of a corrective therapy for an Emotionally Suggestible individual is:

| I | WANT | TO | LOSE | WEIGHT |
|---|------|----|------|--------|
| Woman | Desire | | Frustration | Embarrassment |
| Female | Lacking | | Indecision | Uncomfortable |
| Sexual | Want | | Conflict | Inhibited |
| Frustration | Gratification | | Pain | Insecure |

An example of a corrective therapy for a Physically Suggestible individual is:

| I | WANT | TO | LOSE | WEIGHT |
|---|------|----|------|--------|
| Woman | Need | | Loss | Ugly |
| Daughter | Belong | | Without | Obese |
| Sister | Personal | | Deprived | Unattractive |
| Lover | Self | | Rejected | Unfeminine |

It is important that the client concentrate on one word at a time and what it means to him so that he loses the concept of the sentence as a whole, while he works with the parts. The original sentence represents the conscious interpretation of the feelings; the synonyms represent the symbols brought up by the subconscious mind. Each word represents another step deeper into the subconscious mind because, whenever the conscious mind becomes taxed (as it will, while trying to think of a series of synonyms), the subconscious mind takes over. By the time he reaches the end word, the client is reaching the feeling of what the first word really means to him. The last sentence of the corrective therapy is, therefore, the most important. The other sentences can be used as clues to behavior, especially if the cause is superficial, but they serve mainly as misdirection, in order to allow the true subconscious symbols to emerge.

In the above examples, the Emotional female begins to reveal that she is feeling very frustrated, is gratifying herself by eating, and is feeling tremendous pain from the insecure feeling of not having control. The reality of her last sentence represents her feelings of frustration because she cannot control the weight.

The Physical female feels that men will reject her because she is not feminine. She does not really believe that the excess weight makes her unattractive, but fears that men will reject her because they care solely for her body, not her mind.

The last sentence is the clue to the therapeutic suggestions. You would suggest to the Emotional that:

*We are going to eliminate your frustration and insecurity, removing any conflict or pain that may have caused this feeling of loss of control.*

Do not specifically refer to losing weight. This type of suggestion implies that, if the frustration disappears, so will the weight.

With the Physically suggestible subject, you would suggest that:

*Your motivations for losing weight are that men will accept you for, both, your mind and your body, and that by losing weight, you will be doing something good for yourself.*

Corrective therapy is used if the symptomatic approach has caused an abreaction, resulting in an increase of the symptoms, or if circle therapy has not been effective in removing the symptoms.

Once the cause is eliminated, the symptom will disappear, and when the removal of the cause is reinforced subconsciously through repetition of a suggestive idea, the eradication of the symptom becomes permanent.

The client can write out a corrective therapy at home in preparation for his therapy session, just as he writes down dreams to bring in. Corrective therapy gains effectiveness, when used in conjunction with dream therapy to reinforce the subconscious symbols.

## DREAM ANALYSIS

A basic understanding of dream analysis is necessary to properly utilize the natural venting process of dreaming. There have been many books and theories written on dream symbols and numerous experiments conducted on dream analysis. I believe that symbols represent different things to each person, and that dreams deal with the unique subconscious symbols of each individual. Your conscious understanding of a symbol is usually the correct interpretation. A generalized interpretation cannot possibly fit everyone. For example, if you dream of a dog walking toward you, the dog becomes a symbol. If you love dogs and have not had any bad experiences in your life dealing with dogs, it is a positive symbol. For someone who fears dogs, it is a negative symbol. All symbols in dreams deal strictly with you as an individual.

Everyone dreams. You may dream for up to ninety minutes out of an eight-hour sleep period. The depth of your sleep determines whether or not you remember what you have dreamed. The lighter your sleep, the more you will remember. The sounder your sleep, the less you will remember.

There are three types of dreams. Dreams that take place during approximately the first third of your night's sleep are called *wishful thinking dreams*. These deal with events or thoughts of the day that your mind is accepting. This type of dream has very little value as far as dream analysis is concerned.

Dreams that take place in the middle of the night, or approximately the second third of your sleep, are *precognitive dreams*. These are events that your mind predicts will happen. You mind is constantly accumulating information based on what you hear, see, and experience in your day-to-day life; and, sometimes, it expresses its conclusions as symbols in the dream process. Most of the time, this type of dream is lost totally or partially to the memory, and so it becomes difficult to analyze. Should you be awakened in the middle of the night by such a dream, it is important that you record it in writing for future analysis.

During approximately the last third of your night's sleep, venting dreams take place. These dreams are the most important to dream analysis, since they represent events, traumas, doubts, and fears that you are removing from your past and present. They reflect that which you no longer need to hold onto. They must always be recognized and accepted as a venting process, and not be misinterpreted as having precognitive value. The purpose of venting is removal. If you take these dreams back into your mind literally, instead of recognizing their natural therapeutic value, you are not allowing your mind to let go of the condition that it is trying to release.

To understand your dream symbols, you must recognize that there will always be timing clues in a dream, telling you what period of your life the material comes from. For example, should you have a dream where everything appears to be in the present, with the exception of one person you have not seen since you were twelve years old, this clue indicates that you are venting out something that took place when you were about twelve years of age. Specifics of what is being vented will be indicated by the events of the dream. It is probable that the condition being vented has been reinforced by other experiences throughout your life, and, if so, this dream (or subsequent dreams) will show evidence of this by way of timing clues. The timing, then, will indicate if the symbols of the dream are to be interpreted according to a present or a past state of mind. The timing device takes you back to what you are trying to vent and brings it into the present. Some dreams may have unrelated people or places from many different periods of your past. If this is the case, you are venting all the different occasions you experienced a particular condition. A dream will remove the condition it is reflecting, only if it is understood consciously, as based on the symbols and timing devices.

Following are some of the main reasons for using dream therapy:

## 1. Starting the flow of venting, if venting has been blocked.

Dreams are the only natural and complete venting process inherent in the human being; and, as such, they allow us to remove any overabundance of accumulated message units that we have not been able to deal with during our waking hours.

Venting in dreams can be blocked by unpleasant or threatening recurring dreams, fears or phobias, or the misinterpretation of a previous buildup of message units. These conditions throw off the dream cycles that would normally take place because they cause a person to toss and turn restlessly and to wake up many times during the night. Once the dream process has been blocked or interrupted, the buildup of trapped message units in the mind creates an anxiety that progressively builds momentum, eventually giving way to either physical or emotional pain. At this point, dream therapy becomes essential to bring the person back to normal functioning.

### 2. Searching out a cause for symptoms with no obvious clues.

Many causes are elusive in conscious therapy because they are abstract and are derived from symbols. For example, a person who has a recurring dream in which he cannot move his body or talk, and who then wakes fearfully from the dream, may be reflecting a fear of death in sleep; it is the fear that awakens him. The person then exhibits the symptoms of fear of loss of control, when there is no actual cause, except a misunderstanding of the dream.

Another common dream symbol is the act of killing someone. Consciously, it might indicate guilt, fear, or concern about the consequences of killing someone. Subconsciously, though, it might symbolize getting rid of someone in particular only: a dream enactment of the expression, *"I wish he were dead."*

### 3. After the first session, gauging how well your suggestions are working.

Giving suggestions to a client to remember his dreams has a dual purpose. First, it allows you to gauge how well your suggestions are working because the subject will have a tendency to vent out a reaction opposite to your suggestions. In other words, if you give suggestions for confidence, the subject may dream of situations where he had no confidence, thus venting out the feeling of lacking confidence and creating the new feeling of confidence. Secondly, when a client claims to have no memory of dreams before coming into therapy, suggestions that he will dream, not only cause him to remember his dreams, but also reinforce his acceptance of hypnotherapy; that is, the fact that he dreams indicates that your suggestions are working.

## 4. Removing symptoms caused by dreams.

Whenever dreams are taken back into the mind literally, rather than recognized as venting tools, they become powerful suggestive ideas. Usually, when this takes place, the client is in a hypersuggestible state, due to a buildup of message units, which precedes the anxiety state, thereby causing dreams to be real to him subconsciously. If he dreams of a disaster and has no understanding of dreams, he will fear that a disaster will take place, thus increasing the possibility of the formation of anxiety and producing all the symptoms of that fear.

## 5. Understanding the symbols of the mind.

The last sentence of a corrective therapy is a good sample of the symbols of a particular individual's mind. Subconscious symbols are usually created, as the growing child's suggestibility is shaped and developed by events in his life and by the way he is taught to learn. The child goes through many stages of development; and from birth to eight years of age, his subconscious forms many symbols that will continue with him throughout his life. As a person grows up, he will be jogged by his childhood symbols, and, at that time, he will subconsciously relate, not to the present, but to what the particular symbol meant to him at the time he conceived it. That same meaning will be reflected in dreams, as well. For example, if a person has a dream about a gun, and the timing period in the dream is seven years of age, he is venting out a symbol of his childhood, not a reality of the present. If he learned literally, the gun probably represents a toy to him; if he learned inferentially, it can represent what a gun represents to him, such as, the role he was playing at the time or the feeling a gun gives him (power, good, bad, etc.). If a person dreams about a gun, and the dream takes place in the present, it may represent a weapon or the fear of death, according to his current experiences relating to guns.

## 6. Determining when an anxiety is removed.

The dream process will indicate when an anxiety is dissipating, for at that time, the dreams relating to the anxiety will begin to taper off, and the person's sleep will be neither too deep and long, nor too light and short. In addition, he will, of course, feel a lessening of pressure during his waking hours.

## 7. Determining the cause of recurring dreams.

Recurring dreams are the mind's way of trying to remove an event that has been misinterpreted and/or not consciously accepted or understood by the individual. He is refusing, or not able, to release the symptoms associated with that particular dream. Once the recurring dream is analyzed and understood, consciously or subconsciously, it usually ceases to exist. If the dream is misanalyzed, however, it will recur more frequently. Many times, recurring dreams that took place earlier in life cease to occur without therapeutic intervention. This means that the conditions of the dream have been worked out by some conscious process. For example, a teenager may have a recurring dream that he seems to be flying and, toward the end of each dream, he sees himself falling. In this instance, flying indicates the need to escape his present environment, and falling represents a fear of not being able to make it on his own. Eventually, he leaves home, gets a job and his own apartment, and begins to support himself. At that time, the dream will cease to occur because he has resolved the conflict.                    .

As he matures, each human being goes through a series of stages of development and, at each stage he must cast off certain behaviors and adopt others. Whenever his misses a stage of his life due to circumstances that took him away from normal development, he will attempt to relive the events and behavior of that stage through dreams, until he has satisfied the needs that he was unable to fulfill at the appropriate time. For instance, if a person was forced to go to work very early in life, when he reaches a certain level of financial security, he may develop a thirst for knowledge, and his dreams will begin to take him back through his school years. If these dreams develop recurring characteristics, he may attempt to live these events in adult life by, for instance, going back to school to obtain a degree.

### 8. Finding out why certain depressed people do not remember their dreams until they begin therapy.

When a person becomes very depressed, his mind and body, in an attempt to vent out pressure and confusion, have an increased need for sleep. Depression fatigues the brain and the body, causing the person to sleep longer and deeper. If the circumstances that cause the depression do not cease or ease, the person gets to a point where he escapes so deeply into sleep, that he inhibits the dream process and eventually experiences total dream amnesia. If the circumstances that created the depression are eliminated or altered therapeutically, the person's need of deep, long sleep will decrease, and he will begin to vent more and to sleep lighter and remember his dreams. Once this occurs, the dreams can be analyzed as an aid to therapy.

### 9. Understanding how dreams can increase problems.

The most common problem resulting from dreams is the individual's own misinterpretation of what his dreams mean, or incorrect analysis of the dream by the therapist. For example, if a person has a dream where they are reliving an incident where they have treated a friend or relative badly, they may awaken and misinterpret the dream as them being a bad person or having unacceptable desires. This misinterpretation can cause them to re-experience feelings of guilt when in fact the dream was serving as a opportunity to feel, vent and release those feelings and move towards resolution.

### 10. Recognizing how dreams can give false evidence (if being stimulated by a physical condition, such, as, over-eating late at night, drinking, or drugs).

Many times, dreams can give false indications, due to incidents that took place prior to sleep that caused physiological reactions. If a person has eaten very heavily late at night, for instance, he might dream of physical disaster. This is because his body is working so hard to digest the food, he is experiencing physiological activities that would not ordinarily occur during sleep. A frightening dream could also result, if a person became very cold during sleep and experienced a rush of blood to the surface to protect the body temperature. This could cause a fear reaction signal to be sent to the brain, leading to spasmodic shivering of the body and a frightening dream. Further, alcohol or drugs wearing off during the process of dreams can increase inhibition reactions and stimulate dream hallucinations of the fear of loss of control, which can be carried into the waking state as unresolved conflicts.

A good method for gaining insight into how to analyze dreams is to work with a client, until you are very familiar with the way his mind accepts ideas and with the conditions that have affected his life, and, only then, analyze a series of his dreams, interpreting each of the symbols according to his behavior. Then write out a dream that you feel would fit the symbols of this person's behavior. With a little practice, you can predict the type of dreams he will have, by the suggestions you are giving him in therapy.

When you begin a dream therapy program with a client, his dreams will begin to conform to the suggestions you are giving him, and these suggestions will systematically vent out the negative symbols that are in his mind. At the beginning, he will dream out conditions of the past. When he comes to a point where the dreams are all taking place in the present and he feels comfortable when he wakes from his dreams, the dream therapy is over.

*This page intentionally left blank.*

# CHAPTER 7 – HYPNOTHERAPY WITH SPECIFIC CLIENT BEHAVIORS

## HYPERSUGGESTIBILITY AND DEHYPNOTIZATION

A person's individual suggestibility is the way he learns. In other words, suggestibility is the way an individual receives and interprets message units that come to him from within himself and from outside himself. Everyone learns a little differently which accounts for, and is attributable to, the varying degrees and types of suggestibility. *Hypersuggestibility* is a state in which the individual *consciously* responds to his suggestibility, in the same way that he would respond to it in the hypnotic state.

When a person is in the hypnotic state, his receptiveness to what he experiences through his senses, or what he *believes* he experiences through his senses, is intensified. This altered state of consciousness that increases one's receptiveness is, in most cases, blocked from the individual, when he is awakened from the hypnotic state. The hypersuggestible individual's receptiveness, however, is not blocked when he is in the waking state, which means that he experiences the same intensified perception and receptivity in the conscious state that he would in the hypnotic state.

The state of hypersuggestibility is created and triggered by the presence of an overabundance of message units, which cause an individual to attempt to escape this intense input. When these message units become a greater threat to him than the escape mechanism, the individual allows the escape mechanism to take over, as a means of relief from the incoming message units. This offers him momentary solace, but the longer he stays in this state, the greater the chance of permanent hypersuggestibility.

In the conscious state, we have developed survival mechanisms enabling us to curb our senses and feelings, but in the hypersuggestible state, these mechanisms are absent. That is what makes hypersuggestibility such a critical state. It allows the hypnotic state to be a very effective tool for removing hypersuggestibility. Hypnosis is effective in this instance because you can utilize the person's receptiveness to positive changes, without being hindered by his defense mechanisms.

One type of subject who will often require Dehypnotization from hypersuggestibility is the natural somnambulist. Many of them are walking around in an obvious trance state. This type of subject feels so much physically and emotionally and responds so strongly to the environment, he may be capable of developing psychosis as a means of escape from the reality of his problems. Most psychotics are natural somnambulists; but this, of course, does not imply that most somnambulists are psychotic. There is always the danger that a subject with suggestibility other than somnambulistic (who is unable to escape reality through psychosis) may escape into suicide, should the anxiety build to unmanageable proportions. However, it is very unlikely that a natural somnambulist would resort to suicide, for he can retreat into his own world of fantasy.

Since hypersuggestibility is more common among Emotionally suggestible subjects than among Physically suggestible subjects, more Emotionals are apt to require Dehypnotization. Some common expressions you will hear from Emotionally suggestible subjects, after they have been hypnotized and awakened are: "I didn't feel anything;" "I heard everything you said;" "I could have opened my eyes any time I wanted to;" and "I can't be hypnotized." These are conscious, rather than subconscious, feelings brought about by the fact that you affected the client's critical area of mind, simply by the implication that you were going to hypnotize him. A person who says that he cannot be hypnotized really means that he is suggestible to you and is afraid he will be hypnotized. If a person is very defensive and critical, you should tell him before putting him into hypnosis that, when he awakens, he will probably say that he could have moved, opened his eyes, etc. Then, when he does come out and starts to repeat exactly what you predicted, it will shock him slightly and will help break down his barriers. His suggestibility will change a little during the next session because of this.

Many hypersuggestible Emotionally suggestible subjects have

already entered a state of hypnosis before they walk through your door, simply because of their own expectation of entering the state of hypnosis. This type of subject will also be affected by thoughts given before he enters hypnosis. Therefore, before you hypnotize him, always tell him how you are going to induce hypnosis and what areas you are going to work with, once he is in the state. As he is listening, he will probably be thinking that it will not work, but at the same time, he will be taking in everything you say. Since he does not believe he is in hypnosis yet, he does not feel threatened or defensive.

When he closes his eyes, rapid eye movement will take place immediately. This confirms that he is in the state of hypnosis already. Because he did not want you to affect his physical body, he escaped into hypnosis, even before you had a chance to hypnotize him. However, you must go through the formality of counting him in and saying, Deep sleep, so he will believe that his is hypnotized. Once you have done this, he is likely to become defensive because he fears your control; therefore, you should give him general suggestions of well-being only, and then awaken him.

When he opens his eyes, you will see that they are glazed and that he is still very receptive. It follows, then, that what is said to a hypersuggestible subject immediately after he awakens from hypnosis is as important as what is said to him while he is in the state because he is still very suggestible. He does not feel threatened by your conscious suggestions because he feels that he is completely in control. Once he realizes that he is responding to your suggestions, he will begin to recognize that his suggestibility can work for him, and he will fight less.

The Emotional subject tends to have a delayed reaction to suggestions because the suggestions bypass his physical body and affect him mentally, by way of inferred, rather than literal suggestions. Many times, he will not consciously understand the meaning of the inferred suggestions, but the thoughts they convey cannot help but reach his subconscious mind. It can take hours, or even days, before he responds, but if you have given the suggestions properly, the subject will begin to feel all of the effects of the suggestions and will become very receptive to hypnotherapy. If you seem to fail, do not blame the subject; blame your own misunderstanding of Emotional suggestibility.

The Emotional subject is often so hypersuggestible, that upsetting or depressing events of the day or things that have been said to him will affect him after the fact, just as suggestions will while he is in hypnosis. Consequently, by the time he feels the trauma incurred, the cause has long passed, and he has no idea what caused him to be unhappy or depressed. For instance, this type of subject may come in and tell you that he was driving down the street and a car in front of him swerved, just missing his car. He drove home feeling no nervous effects, but the next morning, he woke up feeling shaken for no apparent reason. The Physical subject, on the other hand, would have felt the nervousness at the time the near-accident occurred and would quickly be over it. To remove this kind of nervousness from an Emotional subject, all you have to do is make him aware of the cause. If he is not apprised of the cause, situations such as this may create a confusion that will increase his degree of hypersuggestibility. If he begins to feel what he does not believe he should feel or does not know the cause, he will compound the problem by developing stronger defenses.

During the hypersuggestible state, the body is nervous and anxious, sending many unnecessary message units to the brain. By relaxing the body in the hypnotic state, you can eliminate many of the extra message units and create an association with a relaxed body and mind. In order to prevent a person from remaining in a hypersuggestible state permanently, you must *dehypnotize* him by hypnotizing him, taking him to a depth beyond his present hypnotic state, having him confront and dissipate the conditions causing the hypersuggestibility by means of circle therapy, and then *blocking* his suggestibility so that he will have control of his hypersuggestible tendencies. Whether the subject is in the induced state of hypnosis or a self-induced hypersuggestible state, Dehypnotization is accomplished in basically the same way.

In order to dehypnotize an individual, you must understand suggestibility, how influencing factors work and how the subject is affected emotionally by inferred or literal suggestions. You can prove to the subject that he is in a hypersuggestible state, if you infer certain ideas to him that will produce an obvious emotional response, or if you give him suggestions that will affect him physically at a time when he thinks he is in the waking state. When he feels the effects of these suggestions in the waking state, it increases his belief in the hypnotic state and causes him to be more suggestible to you as an individual.

The mechanics of dehypnotization are as follows: place the subject in a deeper state of hypnosis than he has previously experienced. Suggest to him through inferences or literal suggestions, depending on his suggestibility, that he is no longer suggestible to any negative outside influence, and that his level of confidence will grow. Then concentrate on suggestions relating to the behavior deficiencies that caused his exaggerated suggestibility. For instance, work with his inability to make personal decisions (a trait that usually accompanies hypersuggestibility). Keep in mind also that his tolerance to frustration has been lowered, as a result of too many incoming message units, and that his tolerance level must be raised. Suggest to him that he is becoming calmer and more relaxed and that his energies will no longer be drained by tensions and anxieties developed through indecisiveness and problems of the past. Suggest that he will see things more clearly, that his urgency will disappear, and that he will begin to feel and, therefore, believe, that favorable results are soon coming – for he sees and feels these results in this state.

Then begin circle therapy by explaining to him that he will be doing some subconscious play-acting. For instance, if environmental conditions are depressing him, have him create a mental picture of himself walking outside in the morning and looking up at the sky. The sky is very smoggy, and this really bothers him. He begins to feel depressed. Coupled with depression is a sense of futility. Let him hold onto these feelings for a few moments, then snap him out of it, by telling him that this situation is now in the past. Then give him a series of positive thoughts and ideas, suggesting feelings of well-being and happiness, or any thought that will replace the depression and futility and make him feel better than he did before he went into hypnosis. You might tell him that, each time he is bothered by the smog, he will become aware that it is a circumstance of the environment, that people are doing something about it, and that it is only a minor thing in his life. If he could do something about it, then he would concern himself with it, but since he cannot, he will not let it bother him. He lives in the present, and he has more important things to do today, so he is going to face the smog and be indifferent to it. He will find that, the more he tries to allow it to bother him, the less it will.

Again, have him visualize walking outside and looking up into the smog-filled sky. It will be apparent that it has a lesser effect or no effect on him this time. If his negative reactions have not subsided sufficiently, repeat the process, until they have. Circle therapy can be used to take the subject through any trauma of the past that has created hypersuggestibility or any other adverse reaction.

An important tool used to remove hypersuggestibility and prepare the subject for the blocking process is the Law of Reverse Reaction. In other words, you must constantly challenge the subject in the hypnotic state, by giving him suggestions, followed by reversals. For example, if you suggest that his arm will be stiff and rigid, challenge him, by telling him that the more he tries to put it down, the stiffer and more rigid it will become. Once this potent suggestion has taken effect, repeat the aforementioned cycle, telling him this time that:

> Your arm is stiff and rigid, and you will find that, as you try to bend it, you will become stronger, and your ability to break the influence of suggestions will become easier.

Once the subject is able to move and bend his arm, implant this new suggestion:

> Each time you find yourself in a position where a suggestion is given to you that you feel is detrimental to your well-being, you can immediately command that your mind will be capable

*of greater self-control and will power, and you will be able to break the influence of the suggestion.*

The final step in dehypnotization is to block the subject's suggestibility, to prevent the same conditions from taking place again. This simply involves suggesting that:

*You are no longer suggestible to anything that is against your well-being. You are suggestible only when you choose to enter the hypnotic state and give your verbal consent.*

From this point on, to reinforce the blocking procedure and insure against subsequent hypersuggestible behavior, always ask for the client's consent before hypnotizing him. Finally, awaken the subject, repeating the words, "Wide awake," two or three times to make sure that he is fully awake.

By taking the subject into a deeper state of hypnosis than he has been before, blocking him, and awakening him, you are establishing three very strong conditions that will outweigh and replace his conditioned response to the external environment that has been triggering him into a hypersuggestible state.

## ALTERING SUGGESTIBILITY

Many times, when working with people in therapy, you will find it necessary to alter their suggestibility. Extreme Physical suggestibility is rarely desirable because most people are working with emotional problems that require some Emotional suggestibility, if treatment is to be effective.

If a subject lacks Emotional suggestibility, you must develop it. To do so, create an arm-rigidity, and then add the reversal that the subject cannot bend his arm and that the more he tries, the stiffer it becomes. When he tries and cannot bend it, employ the Law of Association, by saying that, the more he tries, the stronger is the tendency to smile or laugh, or to feel fearful. Even though fear is a negative emotion, it can be used very effectively in cases where a positive emotion does not fit the personality involved. Since the fear will be associated only with the arm-rigidity in this isolated instance, it will not affect the subject adversely or carry over into any other area of his life. Your purpose is to cause the subject to associate a positive or negative emotion with a physical suggestion that strongly affects him, thereby increasing his Emotional suggestibility.

Every so often, you will come across an Emotionally suggestible subject, whose Physical suggestibility must be increased because of the type of problem he wishes to overcome. In such cases, once you have obtained sufficient suggestible depth, you can use the Law of Association to cause your client to associate a physical feeling with an emotional one to which he can already relate. For example, tell him that, in a few moments, when he begins to feel himself smiling, he will find that smiling becomes very contagious. As he is responding to this suggestion, which affects his emotional behavior, suggest that his jaw feels heavy. This will produce a physical response of heaviness that he would not have felt, had it been suggested to him directly, and the physical response will increase his Physical suggestibility.

Because smiling is not only an emotional response, but additionally requires physical movement, it can also be used as a starting point to increase Physical suggestibility by a more direct means. In other words, a person may be smiling inside without showing it. If you believe that this is the case with a client, you can stimulate the physical manifestation of the smile by using a laughing tone of voice. The fact that he is smiling inside forces him to become suggestible to that inside feeling, and it manifests physically as a grin. When this happens, you have affected your client's physical body, thereby stimulating an increase in his receptivity to physical suggestions.

## GENERAL SELF-IMPROVEMENT AND MOTIVATION

Approximately 80% of the clients seeking a general self-improvement therapy are women, and most of these women are in the age range from nineteen to thirty. The relatively few men who seek this type of therapy are usually in the thirty- to fifty-year age bracket.

Candidates for self-improvement therapy will generally come to the initial consultation saying, "I want to understand myself better." Their blanket introductory statement is misleading because these people want sweeping behavioral changes, not just knowledge. They come to therapy because some aspect of their lives is no longer good enough, and they want to do something about it. For example, they may believe that they lack fulfilling relationships, career direction, good communication with others, an understanding of their own sexual behavior, the education they want, a good memory, or the ability to make decisions to cope with everyday living. They may have vocational or financial insecurities, conflicts with their parents or partner, or conflicts stemming from religious beliefs, or it may be something as all-encompassing as feelings of hopelessness (often expressed by the clients as feelings of inferiority or a feeling that time is passing them by). Any one of these reactions, or a combination of them, may cause a person to seek therapy.

On the whole, these are the best clients for hypnotherapy because they take their therapy very seriously and work diligently towards their goals. They are also a good source of client referrals. With them, therapy tends to go smoothly, although major life crises or changes may precipitate therapeutic crises.

A major part of self-improvement therapy involves giving conscious feedback and providing a direction and a series of goals. Self-improvement therapy can be outlined in a step-by-step manner more easily than other therapies. A good working model follows:

*First Session*: Have the clients talk out their problems, telling you everything they can about themselves. If desired, administer questionnaires, especially the sexuality questionnaires. Explain their sexuality to them just enough to show them that their behavior is normal. Explain suggestibility, test their suggestibility; hypnotize them. While they are in hypnosis, give suggestions for feelings of well-being and confidence.

*Second Session*: Initiate dream therapy and suggest that the clients keep a diary relating what they think and feel, between sessions. (This increases conscious participating by the clients and increases their feelings of value and self-worth.) Tell them to bring to the third session a list of all the concrete self-improvement changes they wish to make. Hypnotize them and give suggestions for feelings of confidence and self-worth.

*Third Session* (and following): Have the clients turn in the list of all the changes they want and have them decide which item will be the first to be worked with in depth. The first item must be one with which you can obtain effective results at that point in therapy, but it must not be a minor one. If it is, the clients will lose interest and motivation. Outline a plan to handle the first item, and begin working on it with both hypnosis and conscious discussion. Each week, have the clients indicate how far they have progressed on the target item, based on a scale from one to ten. When ten is reached and maintained, that particular problem is resolved. Continue this same pattern with each of the other target items.

Occasionally, a client will come in complaining that he is completely lacking in motivation, so much so, that he does not even have enough incentive to work toward self-improvement. Such a client is generally forced into therapy by a worried spouse or relative who is distressed by the individual's haphazard lifestyle and emotional and physical inertia. Obviously, such a subject must become motivated before other areas of his behavior can be modified.

Since motivation is purely subconscious and deals with an emotional feeling, you must first instill in the subject a conscious desire for motivation. Some basic clues for accomplishing this with different behavior types are: the Physically sexual, Physically suggestible individual is most motivated by the idea of being successful enough to brag about his accomplishments; the Emotionally sexual, Physically suggestible person has to receive compliments on his successes; the Physically sexual, Emotionally suggestible has to increase his material holding; the Emotionally sexual, Emotionally suggestible is most concerned with earning potential and the power it will give him.

As with the highly motivated client, it is necessary to help the non-motivated individual to set goals – preferably short-range goals – that can realistically be met. Additionally, you must stimulate in his subconscious the feeling he will have when he arrives at those goals. Have him visualize or imagine his goals, as well as experience the feelings he will have, once he has accomplished them. Continue this approach until he is able to associate the feelings with the desire. When he is able to do this, he can truly be motivated to further change and success.

## HYPOGLYCEMIA

This section is included because so many symptoms of hypoglycemia (low blood sugar) are also symptoms of emotional disorders, that the hypnotist can sometimes be confused or misled in cases where hypoglycemia is present. For instance, he may find that the symptomatic approach is totally ineffective for no apparent reason. If this occurs, he should consider the possibility that the cause of the emotional problem lies in a physical condition, such as hypoglycemia.

Low blood sugar takes place when there is an insufficient amount of sugar to supply the energy demands of all the cells that make up the body and its organs. Since the body derives its energy from sugar, it cannot function properly when deprived of it. The tendency to have hypoglycemia can be inherited from either parent, or can develop during gestation. If the mother has low blood sugar during pregnancy, she will draw on the adrenal glands of the child, causing the child to be prone to develop hypoglycemia. The most common causes, however, are physical or emotional stress (especially if strong or continuous), poor eating habits characterized by too much carbohydrate intake and not enough protein, or excessive intake of chemicals, such as alcohol or drugs.

Some of the common symptoms of hypoglycemia are:

1. Irritability, depression, nervousness, anxiety
2. Decreased ability to cope
3. Chronic fatigue or weakness, especially in the morning

4. Inability to lose or gain weight

5. Decreased Physical suggestibility (Whereas a written test may show extreme Physical suggestibility, the active test will show very little.)

6. Feelings of panic or loss of control

7. Headaches

8. Confusion or forgetfulness

9. Difficulty concentrating

10. Difficulty controlling temper and emotions

11. Insomnia, nightmares

12. Tremors and cold sweats

13. Heart palpitation

14. Addiction to coffee, alcohol, cigarettes, or drugs

15. Cravings for sweets and pastries

16. Allergies, asthma

17. Dizzy spells, loss of balance, vertigo

18. Convulsions

19. Blurred vision

20. Itching or crawling sensations of the skin

21. Loss of libido

22. Nausea

23. Muscular pains, leg cramping

24. Gastrointestinal distress

25. Phobias

26. Symptoms of paranoia

27. Nervous breakdown

28. Suicidal ideation

These reactions usually take place after long periods without any food (such as, first thing in the morning), after periods without protein foods, or after the intake of foods with a high sugar content. The more extreme reactions, of course, come about only after long periods of suffering from this condition.

If you suspect hypoglycemia, send your client to his medical doctor or to a hypoglycemia specialist who can administer the five-hour *Glucose Tolerance Test*. Hypoglycemia can usually be controlled by diet. Once a person with this condition has stabilized a healthy pattern of eating, hypnotherapy can be very useful in removing any associations, fear habits, or symptoms that he may have acquired as a result of his physical condition.

## MEMORY IMPROVEMENT

The hypnotic state produces or increases a variety of behaviors that are most helpful as an aid to improving a client's memory. For example:

1. Hypnosis can be used to increase a client's comprehension of, and concentration on, material that is important for him to remember at a later date.

2. Hypnosis can help a client relax, which will enable him to better direct the attention of his conscious mind, while he is trying to study or remember.

3. A client's feelings of personal well-being can be raised in hypnosis, and such feelings are closely related to successful accomplishments in all areas of self improvement.

4. A person's motivation and desire to have a good memory can be increased in hypnosis.

5. Hypnosis can help eliminate a subject's fears about failure to accomplish any goals that he sets for himself.

6. Hypnosis can be used to increase a client's ability to visualize material studied earlier, and this can produce the so-called photographic memory.

7. Beneficial suggestions for memory improvement given in hypnosis will depreciate slower than similar suggestions given in conscious therapy.

When working to improve a client's memory, always incorporate all of these aspects of hypnosis into the general plan outlined below.

You can begin to improve a person's memory, simply by removing some of the blocks of the past and some of the common negative thoughts that have been put into most people's minds.

The major example of such negative injunctions is: "Don't crowd your mind with details and all those unnecessary facts." The human mind is so large that it could not be filled in an entire lifetime, and we are capable of remembering everything we have ever seen, heard, or experienced. We are capable of recalling almost any information we desire to remember – with desire being the key word.

When working with memory improvement, give your subject a series of suggestions to stimulate his desire to remember, making memory a mental game. Help him learn how to exaggerate. Since the mind will accept and never forget exaggerations that have been properly put into it, use a simple, exaggerated visualization, in order to impress upon the client the value of exaggeration for memory improvement, and in order to build his confidence in his ability to remember.

For instance, you might have the subject visualize an orange house on a hill. It has no doors, no windows. On the top of the roof is a thirty-foot flagpole, and on top of the flagpole is a little pennant with a tic-tac-toe on it. Coming down from this pennant is a long silver chain. At the bottom of the chain, a 175-lb. blue cat is hooked. Now, the cat is trying to crawl up the side of the house, and there are little tires all along the side of the house that keep falling off the house and rolling down the hill. The tires roll into a little money tree. Money is falling onto the ground from the money tree, and the client sees himself picking up the money, which has the word imagination written all over it.

The purpose of this seemingly nonsensical exercise will become evident, when the subject is asked to repeat it an hour or a week later, and is able to readily recall every detail because of the absurdity of the overstatement. As a reinforcement, suggest that any time he has the desire to remember anything, he will add an exaggeration to the memory. He will also constantly add to his thought pattern the fact that he does remember, will eliminate any negativity relating to his memory, and will never say to himself, I cannot remember.

Simple suggestions, such as, "Your concentration, your retention, your recall, and your memory, consistently improve," are effective hypnotic suggestions that stimulate the subject's own expectation of memory improvement, as well as his desire and motivation to succeed at improving his memory.

## NAIL-BITING

Nail-biting can be a symptom of anxiety or simply a nervous habit. When it is a nervous habit, the subject is usually not aware that he is doing it. He may bite his nails when absorbed in a movie, a book, a conversation, or his own thoughts; but when it is brought to his attention, he can stop without any signs of upset or anxiety.

If the nail-biting is a sign of anxiety, the individual becomes tense and upset when it is brought to his attention. The anxiety is usually caused by a situation he feels incapable of handling, such as, exams in school, a new job, or problems in a relationship. When nail-biting is caused by anxiety, a replacement must be used. The replacement may simply be the awareness of the rewards of overcoming the nail-biting, or it may have to be a definite material replacement.

Since a nail-biter is usually nervous, a more paternal induction, such as, the arm-raising test, should be used. The only disadvantage of the arm-raising test, in this case, is that the nails are exposed; and if the subject becomes too self-conscious about them, it will slow down the induction. A good induction that avoids this problem is the direct stare induction with a paternal patter.

Generalized suggestion to eliminate nail-biting should include relaxation; loss of tensions, anxieties and pressures, and increased confidence and motivation to quit. It is usually very effective to have the subject visualize or imagine long, clean, attractive fingernails. Sometimes, however, the rewards of longer, clean nails are not a strong enough motivation to act as a replacement. If the subject begins to abreact to this suggestion, it is an indication that a stronger replacement is necessary.

If this occurs, you must take the symptomatic approach and give your client the option of a material replacement, such as, a manicure set, a nail clipper, or other incentives that will promote awareness of the nails and give him something to do in place of biting his nails. A new hobby that requires the use of the fingers or fingernails is a good replacement.

If the symptomatic approach does not work, the cause must be sought out. Probably the most common cause is sibling resentment or a reaction to parental restrictions as a child which has turned into a self-perpetuating form of gratification or fixation. Regression can be used to locate the cause and can then be followed by circle therapy to neutralize the cause.

## INSOMNIA

Sleeping is a habit. Insomnia, or the inability to sleep through the night, can be caused by many things. Quite often, insomnia is attributed to the intake of coffee or tea; hunger pains; noises; a too hot, cold, or stuffy atmosphere, etc. Belief in these causes makes them real to some people, and can actually cause insomnia. However, an inability to sleep is usually caused by an overactive mind, trying to deal with present-day problems, tensions, anxieties, and pains. Just the anticipation of an exciting event that is to take place the following day, will often keep a person from sleeping the night before. But this occasional insomnia is no need for concern because it will cease by itself, once the anticipated event has been actualized. However, in cases where insomnia stems from emotional problems, the emotional problems must be removed before sound sleep can be achieved. Fears of the past, a fear of loss of control, or a fear of death can also cause insomnia.

Often, the individual suffering from insomnia will make the usual, but unsuccessful attempts to overcome counting sheep, drinking warm milk, reading, exercising, vacationing, etc. These are temporary solutions, at best. However, insomnia is one of the easiest of all hypnotic therapies, especially when it stems from tensions or over-activity of the mind. After a hypnotic session, and without any suggestions whatsoever regarding his problem, the subject will usually sleep very soundly and deeply that night because of the total bodily relaxation he experienced.

Of course, direct suggestions can also be given that the subject will sleep quickly, soundly, and deeply throughout the entire night; and when he awakens in the morning, he will be alert and active, with a feeling of well-being. A post-hypnotic suggestion should be given that, each time the subject places himself in a position to sleep and begins a count from 100 backwards to zero, long before he reaches zero, his mind will drift into a very calm state, and his subconscious mind will draw him into the sleep state.

Some appropriate suggestions that can be given consciously, as well as subconsciously, are:

- *Concentrate on relaxing daily.*

- *Eliminate the thought of sleeping or not sleeping.*

- *Pick one comfortable position and stay there until sleep comes, since moving about in bed stimulates insomnia.*

- *Avoid unnatural aids for sleep.*

- *Practice relaxing in the presence of noises or pain.*

The purpose of these suggestions is to make the subject aware of how to replace old conditions and habits with new and positive ones.

## STUTTERING

Generally speaking, a person who stutters is a highly suggestible individual. Stuttering can be caused in such a highly suggestible person by many things, including insecurity, fear of speaking in front of a classroom as a child, domineering and overwhelming parents, identification with others who stutter, rebellion against rigid authority, or simply faltering because of bad pronunciation of words.

The symptomatic approach is the most effective way to work on stuttering with hypnosis. A general patter of suggestions would be:

*You are relaxed. Tensions, pressures, and fears are gone. You are calm and confident, and you cannot stutter or feel hesitation in your voice. Your brain and your speaking voice are in perfect harmony and timing. You speak slowly and deliberately, and even if you try now, you cannot stutter; the more you try, the more impossible it becomes to stutter.*

Next, tell the subject to open his eyes without awakening. Allow him to speak to you for a few minutes. As a rule, a stutterer cannot stutter while in hypnosis. This inability to stutter can be used to create an identification with a new natural state of speaking clearly. If he is able to speak without stuttering, suggest that he again close his eyes and go deeper. Begin to speak with rhythm and strong conviction, confidence, and command:

*Now you have just proven to yourself that stuttering is impossible … because you are relaxed. This relaxation becomes a permanent habit with you, and each and every day, you begin to speak slowly, deliberately, and confidently. You now know that the fear of stuttering is gone, and this new habit becomes very prominent in your mind. You strongly desire to talk effectively, slowly, and rhythmically, and when you talk this way, you are actually thinking out every word and sentence that comes out of your mouth.*

When the subject is in the waking state, have him concentrate on your forehead, or some other point of fascination, while he talks to you. When he does this, his attention is directed away from his stuttering. The more he concentrates on, and becomes consciously aware of, his problem, the more he will tend to stutter; the more he concentrates on something else, the less the tendency to stutter.

A client who stutters may be encouraged to sing or to memorize a speech, since both of these foster development of rhythmic vocalization. It is not advisable to teach a stutterer self-hypnosis, however, because of his high suggestibility, and regression should be used very sparingly, if at all. Of course, always stress the importance of not stuttering, and discuss the many ways in which the client's life will improve, when he speaks freely and without hesitation.

A stutterer should be seen about two times a week for approximately fifteen sessions so that he receives sufficient reinforcement to make permanent his new confidence in his ability to speak properly.

## CHILDREN'S BED-WETTING

It is not unusual for small children to wet their beds. The medical term for bed-wetting is enuresis. Although it is a nuisance, there is no cause for alarm, unless it continues long after the child has reached the age when he can reasonably be expected to stop, or unless a child who has stopped bed-wetting, reverts back to it. This is the time when hypnosis should be used.

There is no specific age at which a child learns to control his bladder. A child will not last the night without urinating, until his bladder is physically large enough to hold a night's worth of urine. Some children are able to control their bladders by the age of three, while others might not learn until five. Some have a small bladder capacity, but are able to avoid bed-wetting because they do not sleep as deeply as others. However, most children are sound sleepers. This characteristic, when coupled with small bladder capacity (usually a heredity characteristic), will result in bed-wetting.

Bed-wetting sometimes occurs when a child has a difficult time adjusting to a new situation, such as, a new baby in the family, starting school, recovering from an illness, or having attention suddenly taken away. Some children wet their beds because they want their parents to visit their bedrooms during the night.

When working with a child on this problem, educate the parents to establish a certain pattern with the child. This pattern involves encouraging the child to drink an abundance of liquid and hold it as long as possible. This will gradually increase the capacity of his bladder. The child, of course, should always go to the bathroom before going to bed. Also, the parents can set an alarm for the child in the middle of the night and gradually extend the alarm time, until he no longer needs to awaken. If the parents take the child to the bathroom, they must be sure that he is fully awake so that he identifies with urinating in the waking state, rather than in the sleeping state.

Before hypnotizing a child, make sure he consciously understands the words you are using. The suggestions given once the child is in hypnosis, should follow this pattern:

> *Each and every time that you have to go to the bathroom while you are sleeping, you will not only feel it, but you may dream of it. You will awaken very quickly and will get up and go to the bathroom. Your bladder will remain tight, until you reach the bathroom. You are very happy that you can control the normal function.*

Children respond quickly and dramatically to hypnosis. The entire process of hypnosis, including physical suggestions, should be like a game that the hypnotist is playing with the child. It is important that a good rapport be established so that the child wants to please the operator, as well as himself. Always end the session with the child feeling or seeing something happy so that he does not become bored with his hypnosis sessions.

## HYPNOSIS FOR PREGNANCY AND CHILDBIRTH

Hypnosis can be very useful during pregnancy and childbirth because the relaxation and control that it produces make for a more comfortable pregnancy and easier delivery.

Hypnosis has many advantages over chemical anesthetics. For example:

1. Hypnosis, unlike some familiar chemical pain relievers, cannot possibly harm the child or the mother. Also, since it is a comfortable and pleasant experience, neither mother nor child will have to suffer the unpleasant side effects often associated with conventional methods. In certain cases, some anesthetic or relaxing drugs may be required, but the amount needed will be greatly reduced, if used in conjunction with hypnosis.

2. The calm, relaxed state of hypnosis increases the resistance to fatigue, while it decreases the degree of shock to the system.

The combination of effects helps to promote a rapid recovery after delivery and a good supply of milk for breast-feeding. Further, the lack of shock and discomfort to the mother will usually pass on to the child.

3. With hypnosis conditioning, the cervix can be made to dilate more quickly and easily so that the early stage of labor can be shortened. In the same way, the muscles of the lower portion of the birth passage can also be relaxed, in order to facilitate the descent of the baby. This increase in muscular relaxation means that there is less pressure on the baby and on the umbilical cord, so damage from compression is less likely to occur. Not only does the child benefit from this relaxation, but the mother's pain during delivery will be considerably reduced as well, since much of the difficulty and discomfort associated with labor is due to muscular tension. Mainly because of this increase in muscular relaxation, labor takes place, not only more easily, but more quickly.

Hypnotic preparation for childbirth should always be done with the consent and supervision of the expectant mother's attending physician. Under the guidance of the hypnotherapist, the woman can begin practicing her conditioning in the third or fourth month – once or twice a day, at first, then three or four times a day in the final month.

For childbirth conditioning, you can use the same approach with both Emotional and Physical subjects, with one difference – in addition to the basic approach, have the Emotionally suggestible woman visualize herself going through delivery feeling relaxed and happy.

Always follow the same pattern during conditioning. Place the woman in hypnosis and suggest that she feel a tightening in her legs. When she feels this tightness, suggest that she is letting go and feeling relaxed. Then move her concentration to her thighs and hips, again suggesting that she feel tightness. When this occurs, suggest relaxation of that part of her body. Continue this procedure throughout her entire body, until she can feel pronounced reactions to suggestions of tension and relaxation. Concentrate especially on the muscles of the pelvic and lower back area, which are so important in delivery. Once the tension/relaxation procedure is working smoothly in your office, have your client begin practicing at home.

During your client's hypnotic sessions, it may be helpful to have her choose a physical key word to which she can relate (as in self-hypnosis). Say this key word when you suggest relaxation (but never when you suggest tension), in order to build an association between the word and the total release of tension. Have your client enlist the aid of her obstetrician, by having the doctor say the physical key word during office-visit practice sessions and later during labor and delivery. If, during labor and delivery, the woman says her physical key word over and over, and if her doctor also does so, this will trigger all her past conditioning. If she feels any severe pain, saying her word and concentrating on relaxing the painful areas will provide relief.

The relative ease of childbirth with hypnotic conditioning will be surprising to many women. The conditioning process described is a very natural process of association, and constant practice will increase the expectant mother's belief that she can greatly reduce pain and discomfort during childbirth. This belief will be most strengthened when she feels the full relaxation that follows the release of tensions, when the physical key word has been used. This confident belief in the end results will additionally help remove the fear of pain; and this removal is crucial to developing a tolerance for pain.

Occasionally, a woman will come in during a second (or subsequent) pregnancy, and will say that her earlier delivery was so traumatic that she cannot face the upcoming one. In this situation, desensitize the woman to the earlier trauma by using circle therapy. When the unpleasant residue of the previous traumatic delivery is eliminated, create an association between the now unfrightening earlier delivery and the upcoming delivery. Also develop associations between feelings of pleasant, comfortable relaxation and the current pregnancy, and follow through with the standard procedures detailed above.

When a woman has conditioned herself through hypnosis to remain calm and relaxed during the various stages of labor and delivery, she will be able to control her fear and pain and direct her attention to the birth process itself. When the final dramatic moment of birth arrives, she will experience a thrill of continuity and fulfillment that would not be possible, if she were out with a chemical anesthetic.

## FEMALE SEXUAL DYSFUNCTION

Sexual dysfunction, in both men and women, is a difficult area to work with because the causes of it often lie far back in the person's life. Because of this, the causes of sexual dysfunction are both relatively inaccessible to the conscious mind and relatively resistant to change. Such long-forgotten causes can be a poor or inappropriate handling of the child's sexual questions in the earliest youth; an overly strict or punitive religious upbringing; severe or unwarranted punishment for genital play or toileting accidents in childhood; or parental role-modeling, in which the child is implicitly and/or explicitly shown that sexual expression is *dirty* and *disgusting*.

If a woman has had any of the unfortunate experiences above, she is likely to be unable to achieve orgasm regularly, or at all, without treatment. For obvious reasons, women do not have a physiological inability to have sex, as do impotent men. A normal woman can be *physiologically* ready very rapidly, and can satisfy her partner, but she may not be *emotionally* ready, and may not achieve satisfaction herself.

In some cases, a woman's sexual problem can be at least partially eradicated by a discussion of Emotional and Physical sexuality and a quick overview of normal sexual behavior for her. Generally, however, the problem is more resistant and necessitates a more complex approach.

Masters and Johnson first recognized that all human beings go through the same four stages in each sexual encounter. These are:

1. *Excitement* – in which the individual's thoughts turn to sexual involvement and he or she becomes physically aroused.

2. *Plateau* – in which close physical contact is maintained and sexual tensions reach a high point.

3. *Orgasm* – in which the sexual tensions are discharged.

4. *Resolution* – in which the body and its functioning return to the normal state.

The major difference between Emotionally and Physically sexual females, in relation to these stages, is that the Physical can be ready to participate sexually again within moments after the orgasm and can reach repeated orgasms. The Emotionally sexual woman generally wishes to end the encounter following orgasm (or the plateau stage, if she is unable to reach orgasm) because further contact past that point becomes irritating to her.

Although the Physical female experiences greater sexual release more often than the Emotional, both can develop similar functional problems. If a woman is unable to reach orgasm, it is necessary to elicit the cooperation of her partner for a series of retraining exercises to be conducted at home. Instruct the woman and her partner that, for a specified period of time each day, the man should touch and caress the woman's body, without any inducement to have intercourse and with great attention directed toward the woman's verbal and non-verbal responses to such loving attention. This should be done for a week or two, and these *pleasuring* sessions should be well separated in time from any actual coitus. The purpose of the exercise is to allow the woman to experience pleasurable sensations, without feeling pressured toward intercourse.

Once the woman feels greater bodily warmth and sexual arousal, the man should be instructed to bring her to orgasm by clitoral manipulation. This way she will know what to expect of her body and will be more relaxed as a result of such successes. Ultimately, of course, she and her partner will engage in mutual *pleasuring* before intercourse; and with the pleasant associations of the practice sessions behind her, she will be able to reach orgasm in coitus.

While these practice sessions are going on outside of hypnosis, there is a great deal to be done in the hypnotic sessions themselves. If you are working with a Physically sexual female, have her visualize or imagine the training sessions while in hypnosis. Once she does so, give her direct suggestions that, just as she can be aroused (and, later, brought to orgasm) in the practice sessions, so can she be aroused and brought to orgasm by sexual intercourse. Strong, positive, visual imagery can be used, suggestions for relaxation may be helpful, and systematic desensitization can be used, if the cause of the dysfunction is known.

The approach with the Emotionally sexual woman is different. With her, you must find out why she is unresponsive, and then alter her response to the cause by inferred suggestions and systematic desensitization. The most common reason for sexual dysfunction in an Emotionally sexual female is present-day confusion and misunderstanding about her sexual being. This generally has childhood roots. If the childhood causes are known, they can be systematically desensitized. Then you must work to build up the Emotional female's image of herself as a sexually responsive female and as an individual. Explain to her that the men with whom she shares a relationship are not interested in her sexually alone, but that sexual communication (when it does occur) is as important as intellectual and emotional communication. By building her image of herself as an individual who has (and has a right to) a sexual side, you will enable the Emotionally sexual female to become more responsive to her physical being, which will ultimately result in greater sexual satisfaction.

When working with sexual dysfunctions, it is generally beneficial to have the client's partner sit in on selected sessions, especially if suggestions are made for alternate approaches to sexual fulfillment.

## MALE SEXUAL DYSFUNCTION

Male sexual disorders can range from simple embarrassment to total impotence. The more severe reactions (premature ejaculation, impotence, and *ejaculatory incompetence*) usually have bound up with them some of the lesser problems; that is, the impotent male may be easily embarrassed sexually, may have fears about performance or loss of masculinity, may not understand his sexual behavior, and may experience headaches or muscular pain because of conflicting feelings about sex. Therefore, it is very important to know all of the related complaints a client has, in addition to his presenting problem.

The common childhood causes for sexual disorders listed in the preceding section on female sexual dysfunction also apply to males. Generally speaking, most of the sexual problems that the Emotional male faces are caused by his present-day misunderstandings of his behavior and his need to avoid facing his distressing symptoms. With the Physically sexual male, the main cause is rejection.

When the Physical male is rejected, his desire for sex increases. If he is consistently rejected by one partner, he may not be able to perform with someone else, until he is able to rid himself of the rejective idea created by association with the earlier partner. If the Emotionally sexual male is rejected by one partner, he will be not aroused by that particular woman, but will respond sexually to other women. If the Emotional male has been severely rejected by a woman, it is unlikely that he will ever interact sexually with her again because he resents the rejections, resents the person who rejected him, and punishes that person by his infidelity.

The basic approach to working with male sexual problems is similar to that used with women: A conscious explanation of Emotional and Physical sexuality (especially of their own particular sexuality); re-education and retraining, as necessary; suggestive therapy; and systematic desensitization of cause by means of circle therapy, if this is warranted.

Because of the Emotional male's tendency to avoid facing his symptoms (many times, by avoiding sex altogether), suggestions to create visual imagery, in which the man sees himself performing properly and without anxiety, can be a very effective means of modifying the symptoms. If an Emotionally sexual male is partially or totally impotent, for example, have him visualize sexual encounters in which he is mentally aroused and emotionally willing, and in which he establishes and maintains a full erection. This sets up a strong association between mental arousal (of which he is capable) and physical arousal (which he is trying to achieve).

When working with an Emotionally sexual male who is troubled by premature ejaculation, have him visualize or imagine reaching orgasm at the same time that his partner does. Also have him visualize closing his eyes very deliberately at the point of ejaculation. This association will help the client retard his release until the time that he deliberately closes his eyes.

In an Emotional male, inability to ejaculate intra-vaginally (ejaculatory incompetence) is usually caused by the fear of getting a woman pregnant and the ensuing responsibility of having children, or by overcompensation for a prior experience with premature ejaculation. To work with this problem, have the Emotionally sexual male create a mental image of being *overly* stimulated by his partner, so much so, that he ejaculates after a period of very arousing intra-vaginal containment. This creates an association between sexual arousal (of which he is capable) and coital ejaculation (which he is trying to achieve).

With a Physically sexual male, the approach to alleviation of symptoms is to simply give him direct suggestions to the opposite of his disorder. For example, if his problem is impotence, you can create an association between mental and physical arousal, by giving a literal suggestion that his thoughts will not drift from the sexual experience, but that his mental arousal will elicit physical arousal, resulting in an erection. Suggest that, once he achieves an erection, he will become even more mentally aroused – and, therefore, more physically aroused.

When a Physically sexual male is troubled by premature ejaculation, suggest to him that, each time he penetrates his partner, he will concentrate only on satisfying her. His thought will drift every time he approaches ejaculation, and he will release only when his partner reaches orgasm. As improvement begins to take place, suggest that, next time, he will have even greater control. Continue this until the client is able to satisfy his partner on a regular basis and to control the timing of his own release.

Ejaculatory incompetence is uncommon among Physically sexual men. When it does occur, however, it is extremely difficult to work with because its roots, in most cases, lie in the religious injunction against *spilling the seed* (ejaculating) for any reason other than procreation. The most effective approach to this problem is to hypnotize the client and suggest that he fantasize a sexual encounter. As he fantasizes the desire to ejaculate, suggest that he need not feel guilt over this normal process, but may release his sexual tensions. The association between the desire to release tension, the approval of this action by an authority figures, and reinforcing hypnotic suggestions, will enable the client to complete the sex act.

As mentioned in the article on female sexual dysfunction, it is generally beneficial to have the client's partner sit in on selected sessions, when working with sexual problems, especially if suggestions are made for alternative approaches to sexual fulfillment.

## SMOKING

The two main reasons for smoking are *identification* and *replacement*. In identification smoking, a person smokes because someone he looks up to smokes or because some group he wishes to join contains many smokers. If identification smoking continues after the smoker has ceased to identify with the original person or group, it has clearly become a deeply ingrained habit. Replacement smoking occurs when the individual uses smoking to replace either an earlier habit, such as, overeating, or some deficit in his life (lack of love, companionship, confidence, etc.). A replacement smoker does not smoke simply out of habit, but for the oral and visual gratification – and more for the visual than the oral. He would probably find it difficult and unsatisfying to smoke in a dark room because he could not see the smoke. He receives as much pleasure from lighting and handling cigarettes, as from actually smoking them, and makes almost a ritual out of taking the cigarette out of the pack and lighting it. The truly addicted smoker is a replacement smoker.

Identification smoking is more common and is easier to overcome. The fourteen-day method is used for this type of smoker. Always explain this method to your subject, both, consciously, and subconsciously, as follows:

*Smoking is both physical and mental, so we must change your physical reaction and mental attitude toward smoking. We will start by suggesting that, during the first seven days, you will have an increase in cigarette taste in your mouth. Then, during the second seven days, you will break your cigarettes in half. By smoking both halves of the cigarettes, you will experience heat up to 140 degrees in your throat, mouth, and tongue, causing your chemical reaction to cigarettes and smoking to change. The fourteenth day is your DUE DATE. On the fourteenth day, you will turn your cigarettes over to me. You will then become an ex-smoker, but YOU MUST NOT QUIT SMOKING COMPLETELY BEFORE THE DUE DATE.*

*You will not have any withdrawals for seven days after you quit smoking. The eighth day after you quit, you may have a slight feeling of apprehension. At that time, I will give you reinforcement suggestions.*

During the first seven days, the subject should have two appointments. In each of the first two sessions, repeat the suggestion that:

*From this moment on, until your first seven-day period has passed, you will become aware of an increase in cigarette taste in your mouth and on your tongue. It is an unpleasant, awful taste. You may find yourself cutting down, but YOU WILL NOT QUIT SMOKING UNTIL AFTER YOUR DUE DATE.*

An alternative approach is to use the same basic procedure of the fourteen-day method, with these exceptions: have the subject start the first week smoking twenty cigarettes per day and gauging himself so that the twenty cigarettes last the entire day.

He must smoke all twenty, no more and no less.

The second week he smokes fifteen per day, and the third week, he cuts down to ten per day and changes brands. He takes his ten cigarettes out of the package and carries only them with him all day. He plans ahead of time when he will smoke each of these cigarettes. After he has changed brands, he may smoke less than the suggested number, if he wishes. But before that, he must smoke exactly the designated number.

The following week, he cuts to five cigarettes per day, following the same routine, and then to three per day. He may smoke those three cigarettes no sooner than one hour after meals. His due date will be after he has reduced to three cigarettes for seven full days. This slow decrease in cigarette use helps the person to gradually eliminate the need for smoking and, usually, by the time he reaches ten cigarettes per day, he does not even want that many. However, he must not totally quit until he has completed the entire process.

Suggestions in this gradual reduction method are similar to those used with the fourteen-day method and involve constantly reinforcing the client's goal and suggesting that he does not want to smoke any more (while avoiding the suggestion that he does not need to smoke). The most crucial times in this smoking therapy are the first week, the day he switches brands, and one week after he has quit smoking. This method is most effective, if you can see the person every week until the due date and have a reinforcing session, after he has been without cigarettes for eight days.

If the reason for smoking is *replacement,* a different approach must be taken. A replacement smoker must, at first, be given a replacement or substitute for smoking. A replacement might be something that makes him feel emotionally and physically stronger, such as weightlifting, bodybuilding, jogging, a new diet, or a new hobby. You may also substitute more directly with another habit, such as gum-chewing or drinking coffee, water, soda or milk. The secondary habit will diminish in strength when the original habit is completely gone, so the substitute is actually only a temporary one.

In replacement therapy, reinforcement suggestions for physical and mental well-being should be repeated over and over again. Never mention the harm smoking does, but, rather, the improvements to be gained by giving it up. You may wish to use suggestions revolving around the bad taste of cigarettes. If so, tell the subject that the bad tastes will be eliminated, once he has quit smoking. The habit of smoking for a replacement smoker can be eliminated in just one session, or it may take as many as four or five reinforcement sessions, each identical to the one before.

After a person quits smoking, the old habit will still remain as a conditioning force until his new habits take over completely. When this happens, he will say, "I used to smoke, but I can't even remember now how it tastes." His new conditioned response (not to smoke when the old stimuli are present) has taken over and replaced his old habit.

Many times, clients request self-defeating trade-offs when they are in smoking therapy. A common one is the request to be given permission to smoke filtered cigarettes, instead of their usual non-filtered ones. In such cases, it may bolster the client's motivation to quit, if you give him a few facts: Filter cigarettes give a smoker peace of mind, by allowing him to weaken his fear of cancer through rationalization, but he still sucks in nicotine. Filtered tobacco smoke contains *carbon monoxide* (as in auto exhausts), *hydrocyanic acid* (used in execution chambers), *tars* (used to produce cancer in laboratory animals), *nitric acid* (used to test gold, when mixed with hydrochloric acid, used to dissolve gold), *ammonia* (used to disinfect toilet bowls), and *formaldehyde* (used by undertakers for embalming).

## OBSESSIVE-COMPULSIVE BEHAVIOR

Obsessive-compulsive individuals are people who expend their energy in exaggerated ways because they are repressing an emotional need to act in other ways that might not be considered socially acceptable. The obsessive-compulsive business person, for example, is driven, ambitious, tense, compulsively exacting in all business matters, and fanatically pushing towards a stated goal within a certain time period. The obsessive-compulsive housewife is the woman who cleans between her floor tiles with a razor every day; who becomes anxious or depressed if she cannot clean her toilets daily by a certain time; and who follows her guests and empties their ashtrays when they contain one cigarette butt.

Many times, obsessive-compulsive individuals are simply looked upon as people who have nervous energy; but their exaggerated drive toward perfection and their tremendous need to sublimate, often make it uncomfortable for those around them. Even though they usually achieve considerable material and social rewards for their behavior, their drive tends to limit their chances for personal happiness, and they usually do not function well in marital relationships. Many come into therapy just as their relationships are breaking up, and others come in when they themselves are threatened by their own behavior – when they realize the relative insignificance of sparkling fresh toilets or the corporate presidency by forty, compared with their own peace of mind and a true understanding of themselves.

Following is a list of traits common among obsessive people. In actual practice, the presence of these traits will serve only to confirm your initial suspicions, since the obsessive-compulsive is easily recognized by his driven behavior:

1. Does not live for now, but for a future goal.
2. Is negatively affected by anything that may prevent him from reaching his goal.
3. Has a strong feeling that he will be depressed and, therefore, has a tendency to eat too much, smoke too much, have too much sex, or work too much now, to make up for the hard times anticipated later.
4. Has a fear of death.
5. Usually has additional phobias that stem from his fear of death.
6. Has little interest in people – except to the extent that they can help him achieve his goals.
7. Becomes easily addicted to bad or good habits.
8. Has a tendency toward Emotional suggestibility.
9. Usually has a bad temper.

10. May engage in ritualistic compulsive behavior, such as hand-washing, step-counting, etc.

The obsessive is difficult to work with in a counseling situation, partly because of his inability to form the necessary self-appraising relationship and partly because he is so highly rewarded by our culture for being the way he is. However, there are things which can maximize your effectiveness with such a client.

The best type of induction is a nervous induction, such as the inferred arm-raising, since this will enable you to use this client's normal tension for his benefit. Attempt to increase this client's Physical suggestibility as much as possible. The obsessive's Emotional suggestibility, in combination with his driving ambition, may occasionally combine to form undesirable paranoid features.

To work with an obsessive-compulsive individual, you must first accept his behavior, and then slowly move toward change. Change is realized by uncovering the emotional repression and by integration of valuable life priorities, without loss of the drive for success. You must help the obsessive to live for the present – that will be the most valuable lesson for him. Use the symptomatic approach in conjunction with dream therapy (after you have located the cause), in order to increase self-awareness and alter behavior. Avoid teaching this client self-hypnosis or giving him a tape because he will overuse both and will only reinforce his old behavior patterns. Avoid any type of encounter. Let his change be a gradual unfolding.

People with obsessive personality traits usually require extended therapy sessions to work through and alter their behavior patterns. Such a behavior pattern is deeply rooted, firmly embedded, and highly rewarded in our society.

## FEARS AND PHOBIAS

Fear reactions are primary motivating factors that cause people to seek therapy. Throughout our lifetime, we face situations and circumstances that could, under the right circumstances, create a variety of rational and irrational fears. Most fears have their origin in childhood because the child's limited reasoning ability makes him especially receptive to developing fears of the unknown. (Virtually everything is unknown to him.) This is not to say that fears cannot start later in life due to traumatic experiences of physiological reactions, but most of them have some tie to childhood experiences.

Seldom will you find a person who has a single fear only. Where one fear is present, there are usually many associated and inter-related fears accompanying it. Some of the fears commonly expressed by clients are fears of flying, heights, losing, failing, rejection, pain, exposure, poor performance in sports, public speaking, responsibility, sexual performance, homosexuality, the unknown death, contamination, blood, animals, impending danger, water, the dark, open spaces, closed spaces, and loss of control.

Some fears, such as the fear of death or of impending danger, are, to some extent, common to almost everyone. Others, such as the fear of dogs or blood or the dark, develop out of special personal experiences. If a fear makes a person cautious, it can serve a useful purpose, but if it creates irrational and intense behavior, it interferes with comfortable living and becomes a threat to the person's well-being. A fear becomes a phobia when it reaches the point of being triggered by irrational and unknown factors and when it is experienced often enough to disturb a person's everyday life. People with phobias react uncontrollably and unreasonably to the situation they fear because they do not understand the repressed conflict that causes the intense reaction. It is what the fear represents as an unknown danger, and not just the fear itself, that creates the phobic reaction to it.

In neurotic individuals, a wide variety of exaggerated fears and phobias can exist. Many of the phobias have been given special names, including:

Acrophobia ......................................................fear of heights
Agoraphobia....................................................fear of open places
Claustrophobia.................................................fear of closed places
Hematophobia ................................................fear of blood
Mysophobia ...........................fear of dirt or contamination

Nyctophobia ....................................................fear of the dark
Xenophobia ...................................................fear of strangers
Zoophobia.........................................................fear of animals

Fears and phobias are often created and magnified by the workings of the Law of Association. If, for instance, a person experiences a hazardous and frightening situation, he may become terribly afraid of that specific situation and he may also begin to fear elements incidental to the original event. More specifically, a child who has been in a small airplane during a thunder storm may develop a fear of flying in small and large airplanes, as well as fear of storms, loud noises (from the thunder), men in uniform (the crew), or even what he was eating on the plane. These fears, which may or may not develop into phobias, are carried forward into his adult life. It is interesting to note that, although many people may have been in a situation where an identical threat was present, only some of them will be suggestible enough to the threat to develop a fear reaction.

Some fears, on the other hand, are caused by physiological or chemical problems, such as, a hypoglycemic reaction, indigestion that is believed to be a heart attack, severe physical pain, etc. Most fears originating in adulthood are brought about by association with such physiological manifestations. For example, let us say that an individual is planning to do a lecture in front of a business group. He prepares his lecture the evening before, awakens late the next morning, and rushes to arrive at the lecture hall on time. Her skips breakfast, almost has an accident on the freeway, and arrives at the lecture feeling nervous and upset. As he begins his presentation, he notices that his hands are trembling and that he feels nervous. This could be a reaction to the lack of sugar in his system, or a reaction to the narrowly averted accident; but because the present situation is the lecture, he begins to associate the nervousness with the lecture. Moreover, he may be embarrassed by the thought that someone will see him trembling. Ultimately, he convinces himself that he is afraid of speaking to groups. He may attempt to suppress the fear (which could cause it to grow even worse), but physical trembling now becomes closely related, in his mind, with speaking in front of a group. His association of physical responses to unrelated incidents has created a fear of public speaking.

You can determine whether a fear reaction is physiologically or psychologically rooted, by its duration under the triggering circumstances. In this case, if the cause were physiological, the reaction would intensify, rather than diminish, during the course of the lecture. If the cause were psychological, it would be based on the expectation of the lecture so that, once the speaker became involved in what he was saying, he would become more comfortable and the fear would dissipate. Even though he had physiological reactions during the psychologically initiated response, the origin of the reactions would still be known to him. During a physiologically induced reaction, however, the cause is not consciously recognized and can be improperly associated and interpreted by the individual involved.

Every human reacts physically, as well as emotionally, to the approach of a real danger (storm, automotive, accident, etc.) The physiological changes affect the muscles, nerves, organs, and chemistry of the body, in order to prepare the individual to combat the peril. When the crisis is over, the accelerated pace of the body systems slows and the individual gradually returns to a state of rest.

A phobic person is threatened by something that does not, in reality, pose a life threat. In response to this crisis, the phobic individual undergoes the same emotional and physical accelerations that occur in a real danger situation. Here, however, there is no way to work off the changed state and return to rest because phobic reactions are in the mind and have no basis in reality. Therefore, the phobic person remains in constant turmoil because he is constantly being reminded of his phobia, in that he is always anticipating and dreading the phobic reaction. This turmoil perpetuates more turmoil, so he is never able to confront the fear in a calm state. He, therefore, does everything he can to circumvent it. It is of utmost importance to remember this because it is a rationale behind the hypnotherapeutic use of systematic desensitization to dissipate fear reactions.

# CLINICAL CONSIDERATION OF SPECIFIC FEARS

Many specific fears are an outcome or extension of the *fear of impending danger*. This is a state characterized by a general feeling of anxiety and panic, which is occasionally funneled into one specific fear, but is more often manifested as a foreboding about upcoming disasters from unspecified sources. When based on faulty or irrational interpretations of actual events, rather than on logic and fact, the fear of impending danger becomes a strong neurotic reaction. Whenever the mind subconsciously acknowledges impending dangers that are not consciously perceived, the individual will be thrown into a state of turmoil. He may attach his fear to one specific source, but is more likely to be swept along by a variety of fears, which he believes threaten his destruction. A fear of impending danger is, sadly, common among young children, especially when the parents do not consistently reassure the child, grant him his basic needs, and give him love and security.

**Some of the symptoms of the fear of impending danger are:**

1. High degree of Emotional suggestibility (80-100%).
2. 70% or higher Emotional sexuality.
3. Exhibiting strong abreactions, when tested for Physical suggestibility.
4. Tending to create a conscious panic to avoid physical contact that could be painful.
5. Feeling confident as a driver but not as a passenger in a car.
6. Fearing anything that penetrates the skin.
7. Protective of skin at joints because of thinness of skin.
8. Tendency to be obsessive.
9. Tendency to not trust people easily.

The fear of impending danger seems to have two distinctly different causes. In the first, a person interprets a traumatic dream literally, and then loses conscious memory of the dream itself so that he associates all the events of the dream with the subconscious physiological and psychological experience that occurred during the dream. In the second, a purely physiological or chemical reaction (such as a hypoglycemic attack) takes place in the body without the person recognizing the source. This causes the message units going to the brain to become threatening and triggers the mind to respond irrationally.

*Fear of flying* and *fear of the dark* are two of the most frequently encountered fears. Because any one bit of information could be vitally important in the process of systematic desensitization, all of the information gathered on these two fears is presented below in a checklist format.

## The Fear of Flying could have any one, or any combination, of the following causes:

1. Bad experience on a plane in childhood or adulthood.
2. Bad experience with carnival rides or playground swings.
3. Bad dream experience of the body flying with no control.
4. Falling from crib or being dropped or swung around as a child.
5. Being involved in a car accident.
6. Seeing a frightening movie.
7. Extension of the fear of impending danger. (When a person becomes financially or emotionally successful, he may develop a fear that the good will end and, consequently, he will fear anything that could jeopardize his success).
8. Association with divorce in his family, when one parent leaves by plane.
9. Experiencing air sickness.
10. Unpleasant physical feelings that are associated with a flying episode, such as a thunder storm or loss of visibility due to heavy fog or clouds.
11. Reading a newspaper or magazine article about hijacking or a plane crash.
12. Guilt feelings about taking a vacation.
13. Unfamiliar sounds in an airplane.
14. Restricted feeling related to being tied in by a seat belt.
15. Association with another fear.
16. Superstition.

## Symptoms of the Fear of Flying include:

1. Fear of having no control over the plane.
2. Fear of air-sickness.
3. Fear of panic and embarrassment about that fear.
4. Fear of landing.
5. Fear of takeoff.
6. Fear of air turbulence.
7. Expectation fear before flight.
8. Fear during flight only.
9. Fear of hijacking.
10. Isolation fear, when nothing can be seen below except clouds.
11. Fear of long airplane trips but not short ones, or vice versa.
12. Fear of smaller planes but not larger ones, or vice versa.
13. Fear of unfamiliar sounds in the airplane.
14. Anticipation of facing trauma when arriving at destination.
15. Fear of being tied in or restricted by a seat belt.
16. Fear of loss of control.
17. Fear of impending danger.
18. Fear of death.

**A Fear of the Dark could result from any of the following childhood experiences:**

1. Nightmare that caused awakening in the dark.
2. Almost drowning.
3. Awakening from a nightmare with head under blankets or pillows.
4. Awakening in a strange room.
5. Religious prayers (Now I lay me down to sleep … If I should die …).
6. Attending a funeral of a family member or close friend.
7. Hypoglycemic reaction.
8. Being teased as a child by peers, older siblings, or parents The Boogie Man will get you!).
9. Being confined in a dark place with no route for escape.
10. Thunder storms and lightning.
11. Awakened from sleep by unfamiliar noise outside or inside of room.
12. Family attacked while child sleeps (child has fears

about it after the fact).

13. Being disciplined and locked in room, closet, or cellar.
14. Awakening from sleep to hear mother and father arguing.
15. Association with another fear.

## Some of the possible symptoms of A Fear of the Dark are:

1. High degree of Emotional Suggestibility (80-100%).
2. Fear of sleeping in dark.
3. Insomnia.
4. Hypersuggestibility.
5. Fear of drowning.
6. Fear of dark rooms and buildings.
7. Fear of dark people.
8. Fear of dark streets, highways, and alleys.
9. Dislike of dark clothing.
10. Aversion to the confinement of slip-on clothing or constricting clothing.
11. Aversion to wearing dark glasses (confinement of sight).
12. Fear of loss of control.
13. Claustrophobia (possibly only in the dark).
14. Fear of blankets over head.
15. Superstition (black cats, Boogie Man).
16. Fear of physical pain.
17. Fear of long hallways, corridors, caves, or woods.
18. Religious fears (hell, purgatory, punishment).
19. Aversion to movie theaters, but not to drive-in movies.
20. Fear of death, fear of the unknown, fear of impending danger.
21. Indecisiveness.

A less commonly encountered fear is the fear of contamination, or *mysophobia*. To a Physically suggestible subject, this means an illness that will give him physical pain; to an Emotionally suggestible subject, it means that the body will destroy itself and that he will die. The fear of being contaminated by injection or by infected people in the same room is usually created by parents who are overly protective of a child against illness or disease, who suffer from mysophobia themselves; or who are aware of the amount of negligence in the medical practice. This fear is usually instilled in the child before he is 12 years old. As the child grows older, he will usually dislike the parent who created the problem, but will not want to remember why he dislikes that parent or how the problem really started. To protect himself from his fear, he will usually enter a profession that gives him knowledge of how to prevent contamination or a field that involves mental, rather than physical, treatment.

Another aspect of the fear of contamination is a fear of self-contamination by way of hands or fingernails. A person with this fear is likely to engage in compulsive hand-washing and manicuring. This differs from the fear of oral contamination in that dirt can be spit out and the mouth scrubbed out, but the hands and body cannot be scrubbed internally.

Hypnotherapeutic treatment of mysophobia differs slightly from the general treatment approach for fears and phobias outlined later in this chapter, in that you must:

1. Determine the general cause of the fear, since the cause was a continuous learning process and not one traumatic affair.

2. Create at least 20% Physical suggestibility, if it is lacking.

3. Hypnotize the subject by way of an arm-raising conversion.

4. Make the subject aware of how the fear was created, and avoid forcing any visualization or imagination as to how he reacted to the problem.

*Claustrophobia* is the fear of enclosed spaces, particularly small ones. The claustrophobic in an enclosed space feels trapped, smothered, and crushed. His breathing pattern may be markedly affected. Claustrophobia is closely associated with the fear of the dark, since the dark of night can be seen as a smothering enclosure. It is always very important to correctly identify the phobia being treated, since the sufferer will not be helped by treatment of a non-existent behavior. Claustrophobia is occasionally identified incorrectly as a fear of planes or a car phobia, when, in actuality, the phobic is responding, not to these objects, but to the enclosure that the objects represent.

Claustrophobia occasionally begins in adulthood, when the sufferer experiences some trauma in a small space (people trapped in elevators during power blackouts are likely victims). More frequently, however, it has its roots in childhood, when the child may have been locked in a room or closet or may have been the victim of frightening dreams about being trapped. If a child has been shut in a room as punishment, the withdrawal of parental affection becomes associated with enclosure, and claustrophobia is particularly likely to occur.

A claustrophobic frequently does not seem to be able to remove himself from the frightening situation, even when options for removal are readily available. In a closed room, he does not move to open the door; and in a crowd, he does not walk away. This may be attributed to the childhood roots of claustrophobia – just as the child could not reason about the feared situation, so the adult is incapable of reasoning about it.

A discussion of the *fear of the loss of control* has deliberately been saved until the end of the specific considerations section.

With the background that you now have, you will readily realize that the common element in, and a primal cause of, all phobias is the fear of loss of control. The client may specify that he fears the loss of bodily control, emotional control, or life; but whichever he specifies, he fears a cataclysmic and overwhelming personal annihilation. Many times, there will be religion-based fears. A reverent person may be so guilty about something he has done that he will develop a fear of death and the subsequent reckoning.

Man's evolution has seen him move from less control over himself and his environment to more control. Consequently, the fear of loss of control is a very primitive fear. As such, it is characterized by two equally primitive responses: fight or flight. The sufferer may be enormously hostile and angry (fight) or unmovingly passive and lethargic (flight). The fear of the loss of control, ironically, causes its victims to give up control to one extreme or another.

The fear of loss of control occasionally takes place when a breakup in a relationship occurs. At this time, the Physical partner's behavior becomes highly exaggerated, and he is obsessed by the thought that he must hang on. If the emotional pain becomes so severe that the individual can no longer tolerate it, and fears that he will totally lose control, he could take the route of suicide or psychosis as the ultimate flight from the loss of control.

Like mysophobia, the fear of loss of control involves slightly different treatment approaches. Do not use the symptomatic approach because it will not work in this instance. Instead, work on the conscious level, by exploring the client's rational and logical alternatives. Train him to recognize his options and to choose from them. Then reinforce this hypnotically, using literal or inferred suggestions, as appropriate. When the client's immediate anxiety has been reduced, use circle therapy to have him face and desensitize the areas of uncontrolled feelings.

## GENERAL TREATMENT APPROACH FOR FEARS AND PHOBIAS

When dealing with fears in general, you must keep in mind that all fears manifest identical emotional and physiological reactions, and that the condition that created the fear is a threat to the person because it is unresolved. The cause of a fear initiates the reaction to it. The symptoms are manifestations of the cause, or what the client relates to you that he feels. Symptoms are usually apparent. Causes are usually unknown. If the symptomatic approach fails to remove the fear, it is an indication that you must search out the unresolved conflicts. If the symptomatic approach works, however, it could dissipate the effects of the cause and eliminate the need to identify it otherwise.

Exposing the cause will diminish the anxiety associated with the neurotic fear and take it out of the unknown so that rational therapy and rational suggestive ideas can alleviate the symptoms. It is important to note that some of the causes presently producing symptoms could themselves be symptoms of another cause.

Claustrophobia, for instance, could be the cause of a fear reaction; it could also be a symptom of a fear that was caused by an experience unrelated to claustrophobia.

Circle therapy is the primary tool for identifying and desensitizing the causes. Age regression may also be necessary, in some instances, to locate the cause prior to the application of circle therapy. In some cases, when the fear has been totally desensitized, the memory of it can still cause expectation of the fear, but this is nothing to worry about because, when the individual actually encounters the situation, the fear will dissipate.

## DEPRESSIVE BEHAVIOR

Depression is an emotional symptom that affects most of us at one time or another. When depression begins to dominate a major portion of a person's life, however, it becomes a dangerous condition that creates extreme emotional pain and causes a person to take drastic means of escape, such as drug or alcohol abuse, frantic hyperactivity, or total lethargy, seclusion, psychosis, or suicide. Depression is the end result of the repression of unresolved conflicts over which we feel we have no control. When an individual is depressed, he usually feels unable to make decisions because of circumstances that he believes are beyond his control or because of the seeming futility of any decision or act.

Two of the early signals of oncoming depression are anxiety and boredom. Anxiety is a fight mechanism; depression is the flight reaction that is activated to remove the individual from the anxiety state. Boredom is an emotional conflict that is caused by repression or suppression of either anger, guilt, or feelings of futility. Boredom is present at one time or another in everyone's life. However, an emotionally healthy person finds alternatives to his boredom, whereas an emotionally unhealthy person dwells on his boredom until it takes him into depression.

When a person begins to experience depression, symptoms such as feelings of melancholy and futility begin, in combination with a blockage of venting. (Remember that the only complete and permanent form of venting is through the subconscious mind, via dreams or hypnosis.) Blockage of venting occurs when a person ceases to vent through the normal dream process, usually for one of two reasons:

1. People who are depressed will usually have depressing dreams because the subconscious mind is attempting to vent out the negative conditions. However, if they do not understand the dream-venting process, they are likely to interpret the dreams literally or precognitively and, thus, allow the dreams to pull them deeper into depression.

2. To avoid the pain brought out in dreams, depressed persons may purposefully attempt to suppress memory of their dreams. This causes an even greater buildup of anxieties. In either case, the mind becomes like a clogged pipe, and your responsibility as a therapist is to unclog this buildup and allow it to drain, so that positive input can be received.

When a person becomes depressed, the brain starts receiving signals to vent. Since venting is associated in the mind with sleep, the depressed individual begins to require more and more sleep and to awaken less and less refreshed because he is still holding onto the anxieties that took him into the depression to begin with. Effective venting is blocked, as noted above. If the events that catalyzed the depression are not removed, more sleep will result in more depression, and depressive feelings will begin to dominate a greater portion of the person's life. Usually, this lack of energy and drive compounds the depression; and, many times, the individual will resort to artificial stimulants (which actually cause even greater blockage), in an effort to pull himself out.

One of the end results of perpetual depression, is a state of continued hypersuggestibility. This hypersuggestibility compounds the depression because the person becomes overly suggestible and sensitive to everything around him: the weather seems too hot or too cold, sounds are too loud, traffic or crowds are overwhelming, friends are too demanding. The depression increases, as the hypersuggestibility increases, and vice versa.

The clue to removing depression is to find solutions for the person's unresolved conflicts and to cause the subject to vent through his normal dream process. The Physically suggestible subject, who is not as prone to depression as the Emotional, can temporarily vent and ease the pressure by screaming, yelling, crying, or talking to a friend, a therapist, or even himself. The Emotionally suggestible person, however, needs positive alternatives and positive feedback so that, when he begins to vent through dreams, he is venting the true or inferred causes and not just their literal symptoms.

Always point out to the depressed person what his positive options are because options allow a person to survive. There is only one circumstance under which a person will attempt suicide, and that is, when he has lost sight of his options and feels that he has literally run into a dead end.

As severe as depression may seem, hypnotherapy is an extremely effective tool for its rapid removal because hypnosis can reach the subconscious mind so much faster than conscious therapy, thereby allowing for rapid neutralization of conflicts. The Hypnotherapist must be sure that the client has consulted with a Medical Doctor and/or Psychiatrist regarding this complaint. The Hypnotherapist must receive written confirmation that the Doctor is aware of the client's complaint and sees no problem with the client pursuing hypnotherapy for this issue. Once that is obtained, the following guidelines should be strictly adhered to for quick and effective modification of depressive behavior patterns:

1. Unbunch or separate the problems affecting the client. Work with the most painful problem first, giving alternatives and suggestions on how to handle the situation. Follow the same procedure with each problem in order of severity, being sure to deal with each separately and completely before moving on to the next.

2. Thoroughly explain the message unit concept and hypersuggestibility.

3. Neutralize all negative feelings and thoughts that took

place prior to the hypersuggestible state.

4. Suggest that the subject will dream and will remember his dreams, and then follow through with a proper dream analysis program.

5. Relax the subject's body and mind through hypnotic suggestions, in order to prevent the physical need for excessive sleep.

6. Block the subject from hypersuggestibility, following the dehypnotization process.

7. Establish short-range goals and objectives so that the subject can develop direction and feel that he is going somewhere, thereby eliminating his feelings of futility and giving him hope.

8. Give him the feeling that you are working this out together. Tell him that he must be available and that you will be available to work out and handle all problems. It gives him a sense of security to know that he can always reach you, if the depression becomes severe. In effect, allow the relationship between you and your client to be an escape mechanism that substitutes for further depression or suicidal thought or attempts.

## SUICIDAL IDEATION

Someone who has never been affected by a loved one's suicide or attempted suicide may think of the act of self-destruction as a nebulous abstraction. But to a therapist, dealing with a suicidal client is a shocking and threatening experience that can cause feelings of helplessness and self-doubt.

Why does a person consider suicide? Literature on the subject tells us that many people talk about suicide, but never actually attempt it. It is important to be able to separate the serious cases from those who are just talking, in order to determine when suicidal ideation will actually be acted upon.

I believe that suicide is an escape mechanism that is considered when a person reaches such a deep state of futility and despair that he loses sight of his options and his reasons to live (family, friends, etc.). Suicide takes place when the emotional pain becomes so great and so all-absorbing, that it affects all areas of an individual's life. It is not life itself that a person in this circumstance wants to escape, but the pain of reality.

I personally do not believe in the death-wish concept set forth by Freud. I believe that all humans, by the nature of their existence, seek peace and pleasure, and that the suicidal person has a tremendous need to escape the emotional pain of reality. Suicide becomes a justifiable means of escape because a person who is at the point of committing suicide is not able to consider the consequences of death rationally.

I have found in my studies that the real threat of suicide comes from people who have high Emotional suggestibility and cannot fantasize or hallucinate. This prevents them from creating their own reality to escape the pain of their present reality. A highly Physically suggestible client or a natural somnambulist, however, has escape routes available other than suicide – he can escape into his own fantasy world, or even into temporary or permanent psychosis.

Whenever I find a highly Emotionally suggestible subject who talks about suicide, I become extremely concerned; and that client's problems become a grim reality to me. If you encounter such a client, you must recognize that he needs immediate help. There are several things you can do. First, use extensive conscious neutralizing before inducing hypnosis, and give positive directions as to what the client should and should not do. Second, increase the client's Physical suggestibility, in order to give him an alternate escape into fantasy, instead of suicide. Work at relaxing the body. Develop a plan of short-range goals to accomplish, such as feeling better for longer periods of time. Let your client know that you care and that you are with him and that you will be available whenever he needs you. At the beginning, grant him certain special times to call you. Utilize whatever it is that the suicidal client believes in or cares about very strongly.

This can be religion, children, parents, friends, or yourself. Show him that he has a responsibility to himself, and/or to someone or something else, to live. Let him know that it is not fair to subject others to such hurt because of his selfish need to escape.

Working with potentially suicidal clients is difficult, grueling, and nerve-racking, and requires specialized training. Do not experiment with someone's life. If you have not had appropriate clinical training and supervised experience, refer the client to specialists in suicide prevention. Never begin working with this type of client, unless you have a written referral of a medical Doctor and are willing to take the full responsibility and give the time and expertise that will be necessary to complete this therapy.

# ANALYSIS OF THERAPY

The purpose of the Analysis of Therapy chart is to record a brief overview of each case, which can be used as a quick reference to preceding sessions and also as the first step in preparing a case history. It should be used in conjunction with the Analysis of Induction chart.

1. Name of Subject: _____

Age: _____ Sex: _____

2. Hypnotic Traits: _____

_____

_____

3. Problems/Symptoms:

As related by Client: _____

_____

_____

_____

As seen by Therapist: _____

_____

_____

4. Primary Cause: _____

_____

_____

5. Secondary Cause: _____

_____

_____

6. Type of Induction: _____

_____

_____

7. Suggestions given: _____

_____

_____

_____

_____

8. Purpose of suggestions given: _____

_____

_____

_____

_____

9. Post-Hypnotic suggestion(s) given: _____

_____

_____

10. Should Self-Hypnosis be taught? _____

_____

_____

11. Estimated suggestibility: _____

_____

_____

12. Estimated depreciation time of suggestions: _____

_____

13. History and development of complaint (from onset to present):

_____

_____

_____

_____

_____

_____

_____

14. Previous emotional upsets (from childhood to present)

_____

_____

_____

_____

_____

_____

15. Plan for next session: _____

_____

_____

_____

_____

_____

_____

Notes: _____

_____

_____

_____

_____

_____

_____

_____

_____

_____

_____

_____

_____

_____

_____

_____

_____

_____

_____

_____

_____

_____

_____

_____

*This page intentionally left blank.*

# CHAPTER 8 – RELATIONSHIP COUNSELING

## INTRODUCTION

One indication of the increasing acceptance of hypnosis is the recent legislation that has given licensed marriage, family and child counselors in the state of California permission to employ in their work a means of therapeutic intervention that they have been prohibited from using in the past – hypnosis. Yet hypnosis and marriage counseling are terms that very seldom appear together in scientific literature. For example, a scan of article titles under the heading of *Hypnosis in Psychological Abstracts* for the years 1972-74 reveals only one listing that mentions marriage and hypnosis together (in three pages of listings) and no listings that deal with hypnosis and marital therapy. Perhaps this void stems from a belief that the improvement of marital communication processes is not likely to be facilitated in a therapy that places both partners in a trance state, a situation where real communication could not occur. On the other hand, it is possible that hypnosis has not been used as a tool in marital therapy, simply because of uncertainty as to how it might be applied. It seems appropriate then, especially in light of the pioneering California legislation noted above, to explore ways in which hypnosis might be effectively applied in relationship counseling.

In earlier chapters, we have discussed Emotional and Physical suggestibility and Emotional and Physical sexuality in depth. The purpose of this chapter is to discuss how the interrelationship between suggestibility and sexuality will influence the success or failure of a relationship. While studying this material, it is important to keep in mind the basic premise that *suggestibility* is the way we learn and sexuality is the way we perform or act out what we have learned.

About a decade ago, I observed a correlation between reported relationship difficulty and opposing suggestibilities in the partners. I noticed this because, when working with a client for relationship problems, I often felt it was appropriate to see the client's mate alone for a session. If both partners were cooperative, this is what generally occurred. In the first session with my client, I would routinely induce hypnosis as the first step in therapy and, as a result, assess his or her suggestibility type. Next, I would meet with the client's mate. Invariably, the mate required the opposite type of induction to enter hypnosis. For instance, if the client was a Physically suggestible male, his wife or girlfriend was found to be Emotionally suggestible. This was a very significant finding, especially in light of some of my earlier findings relative to suggestibility, summarized below:

1. The way in which an individual receives messages to enter the state of hypnosis parallels the way he receives messages in his waking state. That is, the type of suggestion to which one responds in hypnosis parallels the type of message to which he is most receptive in everyday life. Carried further, the knowledge of whether an individual is receptive primarily to literal or inferred suggestions tells us whether he is most receptive to interpersonal communication phrased in literal or inferred terms. Therefore, if aspects of a person's suggestibility can be altered in hypnosis (as they can), the potential exists to alter aspects of his behavior in daily life outside of hypnosis.

2. Each person tends to *send* messages in the opposite mode in which they *receive* them. That is, Physically suggestible people tend to communicate their thoughts and feelings through inference, Emotionally suggestible persons communicate in literal terms, and balanced persons communicate both literally and inferentially.

3. A person who communicates on either a literal or inferred level assumes that other people communicate to him on that level as well. This assumption on the part of the individual is not a conscious one. Rather, it is subconscious and stems from the way in which an individual has learned to receive and send information, thoughts, and feelings in communicating with other people.

As I worked with more and more couples, I began to observe similarities in the ways individuals described their mates during private therapy sessions. For example, I quite often found Emotionally suggestible female clients depicting their partners in surprisingly similar ways. As their partners came to meet with me, in accordance with my relationship therapy strategy, I also noticed a similarity in their descriptions of their mates.

I began to make notes of the descriptions that different types of clients gave about their mates. Trends, such as the following, soon became observable:

1. Emotionally suggestible women often described their men as wanting to engage in sexual intercourse *all the time*. These women also frequently stated that their partners *suffocated* them with attention.

2. Physically suggestible males tended to view their mates as having a *weaker sex drive* than was desirable. These men often depicted their women as *moody* and *non-communicative*.

3. Emotionally suggestible males described their partners as *always ready for sex* and as extremely *social* people.

4. Physically suggestible women tended to see their mates as *unemotional* and *non-communicative* with respect to sex and social interaction.

These observations clearly tied in with my concepts of Emotional and Physical sexuality in that the Emotionally *suggestible* partner was describing his/her partner as being Physically *sexual*, and the Physically *suggestible* partner was describing his/her mate as being Emotionally *sexual*. Further research verified the obvious implication that a person's type of suggestibility is usually consistent with his type of sexuality. In other words, a Physically sexual person usually has Physical suggestibility, and an Emotionally sexual person usually has Emotional suggestibility.

However, because of confusions in upbringing, or because of emotional, physical, or sexual traumas, a person may alter his/her sexual or suggestible behavior as a defense against re-experiencing past hurts or confusions. He then develops what we call *incongruent* behavior, which simply means that his suggestibility is the opposite of his sexuality. In other words, he is *performing* (sexuality) differently from how he *learns* (suggestibility).

If a person's verbal expression is inconsistent with his actions, this is also incongruent behavior. For example, when a person says, "I agree with you," while, at the same time, shaking his head no, or if he says, "I want to communicate with you," but leans away from you, this is incongruent behavior. Recognition of such behavior by one partner within a relationship is often expressed in such comments as, "My partner dresses very sexually, but avoids sex," or "My partner's body movements and verbalizations do not say the same thing."

Incongruent behavior is one of the notable causes of relationship and personal conflicts because it results in a breakdown of communication and compatibility between partners, and in confusion within the person himself. Even a temporary incongruent behavior pattern can drastically affect a relationship. The most common temporary behavior change takes place during the *honeymoon stage* of a relationship. At the beginning of any relationship, both, the Emotional and Physical partners are more Physically sexual than they would normally be. If, as the newness wears off, the Emotional partner withdraws into his or her normal behavior, and that behavior is extreme, the Physical partner will become even more Physical, as he experiences what he interprets to be rejection. If the Emotional partner's normal behavior is less extreme (and the change is thus less apparent), the Physical partner will feel secure and confident.

Behavioral changes that take place during the honeymoon stage are particularly deceptive, however, because incongruent behavior is not as apparent as it would otherwise be, due to the blind emotions that characterize that phase of a relationship. Also, there is an overabundance of potential levels and areas of communication at that time, arising simply from the fact that the couple has just met and they know nothing about each other, as yet. The tendency of both partners, of course, is to put their best foot forward and try to communicate what they think the other wants to hear.

Typically, a person will be drawn to his natural opposite in, both, sexuality and suggestibility. Even though many people choose a partner for a certain lifestyle, it still does not alter the pattern of the attraction of opposites within those lifestyles. If an Emotionally sexual and suggestible woman in a relationship with her natural opposite suddenly develops Physical suggestibility, she will not only begin to exhibit incongruent behavior within herself, but she will also throw off the balance of the relationship. Unless the Physical partner also alters his behavior (develops greater Emotional suggestibility) to level out the imbalance, the two cannot help but grow apart.

Individuals who normally function with incongruent behavior will also tend to pick their natural opposites – an Emotionally suggestible, Physically sexual person will be drawn to a Physically suggestible, Emotionally sexual partner, and vice versa. Because both partners have the conflict of incongruent behavior within themselves, they are bound to have additional problems, but, ironically, their problems often draw them together. They may also transfer the blame for their problems to children, relatives, working conditions, etc., and maintain the disturbed relationship, with the rationale that it is the environment or social pressures that cause them problems, and not their own interrelationship. In such cases, their children will tend to reflect the family pathology, by exhibiting unhappiness and bizarre behavior.

Since the maximum percentage of suggestibility or sexuality a person can have is 100%, a variance of five or ten degrees in a person with 80-90% of a particular behavior is much more critical than the same flux would be to a person with a more balanced behavior. Therefore, partners who have at least 30% of their opposing suggestibility and sexuality traits will have enough flexibility to maintain communication and balance through periods of stress or change. If they have less than 20%, it is unlikely that their relationship will survive any undue pressure.

The major overall cause of relationship problems, of course, is simply the coupling of an extreme Emotionally sexual and suggestible partner with an extreme Physically sexual and suggestible mate; and the resulting communication difficulties. The three major conflicts that come about as a result of suggestibility and sexuality imbalances are in the areas of sexual and financial disagreements and communication difficulties. If two of the three are problem areas in a relationship, the chances of a breakup are very high.

A thorough understanding of the correlation between suggestibility and sexuality is the foundation of relationship counseling. It is especially important to remember that, although the base sexuality of a person cannot be altered, suggestibility is always subject to change, in accordance with alterations in one's learning and understanding processes or his life experiences. Therefore, by altering suggestibility, you can actually eliminate exaggerations, misconceptions, and defenses that cause incongruent behavior or that cause a person's sexuality to appear extreme.

The first step you must take when dealing with a couple reporting communication difficulty is to assess the suggestibility and sexuality of each partner. This is done, by meeting with the partners one at a time. The couple is then seen together so that the therapist may explain his findings.

Always begin a joint relationship counseling session by describing the basic traits characterizing Emotional and Physical sexuality, as described in Chapter Five. It is a good practice to also have both clients answer the sexuality questionnaires for themselves, and then also from what they believe would be the viewpoint of their partner. Comparisons of the differences in the way they see themselves and the way their partners see them will give you an immediate insight into the major problem areas affecting their relationship.

Next, you must explain the concept of Emotional and Physical suggestibility, in order to reopen the channels of communication between the two. Each partner must be made to understand that the other thinks, expresses, relates, and functions in a way that is different from his or her own way. This understanding is the first step in pulling the suggestibilities of each individual toward a more balanced state. It is also the first step in breaking down their communication barrier and paving the way for improved communication and increased compatibility, even in cases of exaggerated sexuality differences. When explaining opposing suggestibilities, it is best to explain that the suggestibility has to do with the way in which a person receives messages that influence the way he enters the state of hypnosis. For example, you might say to the Physically suggestible partner that:

*You respond to hypnotic suggestions of a literal nature. When you are given messages that tell you what to feel, you take these messages at face value and respond to them accordingly. You are, therefore, most receptive to literal messages.*

To the Emotionally suggestible person, you would say:

*You are receptive to messages of a different nature. You respond to inferred suggestions. These suggestions present circumstances from which you infer the response that is desired. You do not respond to messages of a literal nature the way your partner does.*

At this point, it is helpful to further clarify what is meant by literal and inferred suggestions, by offering examples of the two types of suggestions. It is also recommended that you assure the couple that both types of suggestibility are normal and that neither type is preferable to the other.

You may then introduce the idea that it is possible that the way in which each of them receives suggestions to enter the hypnotic state may parallel the ways in which they receive messages in everyday life and in their communication with each other. This idea is offered as a starting point from which to begin an exploration of their communication patterns. Continue by presenting the concept of communication as a process of sending as well as receiving information, thoughts, and feelings.

To open a discussion of this aspect of a couple's marriage, you may pose the questions:

> Is it possible that, because each of you tends to receive communication in a certain manner, you tend also to express yourselves by sending messages in a similar manner?

Then ask the Physical partner:

> For example, since you respond best to literal messages, do you feel that you tend to express yourself on a literal level, as well?

Next, ask the same question of the other partner, modifying it to apply to an Emotionally suggestible person. Finally, to facilitate a discussion of relationship communication, direct this question to both partners:

> Is it possible that, since each of you tends to send and receive the majority of your messages in a certain manner, you assume that your partner communicates in that same manner, as well? For example [to the Emotional], do you, as a person who communicates primarily through the use of inferences, believe that your spouse also communicates primarily through the use of inferences?

It should be noted, at this point, that the posing of these questions does not seek to find fault with either partner or the couple as a unit. Rather, this process is viewed as another means by which to facilitate a discussion of communication patterns that exist within the relationship.

Therapy may then proceed with the therapist acting as an interpreter between the partners, as they discuss situations that produce conflicts in their relationship. The therapist, in addition to fulfilling an interpreter role, serves as a source of feedback for each partner, in pointing out how he is communicating his messages on, either, a literal or inferred level. This process should go on until both partners demonstrate an understanding of literal and inferred messages. This may be reflected by new ways in which they communicate with each other.

As the couple begins to understand that their suggestibilities possibly influence the communication pattern within their marriage, you may advise them that suggestibility is a trait that can be altered. In relationship therapy, this process is undertaken with the goal of bringing both individuals into a more *balanced* state of suggestibility. As this begins to occur, the poor communication patterns typically displayed by an extreme Physical/Emotional couple begin to disintegrate.

You can then work with each partner on an individual basis, utilizing the procedure for altering suggestibility, discussed in Chapter Seven. This approach has as its basic premise the notion that, if one variable in an observable correlation is changed, the other variable may change as well. In this case, if opposing suggestibilities are changed (one variable), relationship communication patterns (second variable) may change, as well. This is usually seen to be the case. As suggestibilities become more balanced and old patterns of communication disappear, an improved system of communication develops, stemming from each partner's increased ability to effectively send and receive, both literal and inferred messages.

In the actual hypnotic state, suggestions are focused on eliminating emotional hurts, feelings of rejection, and frustrations felt by each partner. For example, suggest to the man that he is beginning to feel very comfortable in his communication with his partner, and instruct him to visualize himself in specific conflict situations, which offer the opportunity to exercise his new understanding of her communication style. Suggest further that he visualize himself communicating effectively with his partner, by seeking to understand her messages, in addition to making certain that his own messages are clear and understandable. This will desensitize the client, with respect to any resentment he may have built up toward his partner. This idea is strengthened with the suggestion that his objective in seeking therapy is to make his relationship work, and that he is involved in a learning process that entails, not only a better understanding of the way his partner communicates, but a better understanding of the way he communicates, as well.

Suggestions may then focus on building the client's confidence in his ability to communicate more effectively. Once resentment has been removed, this confidence may be built up, in the case of the Physically suggestible man, by employing very literal suggestions, such as:

> *You are feeling very confident in your ability to communicate with your mate. You are confident in your relationship. You are putting all the necessary ingredients into this relationship to make it work. You have come to therapy, and you are attempting to understand your partner's style of communication.*

As this therapy is going on with the man, the identical therapy is done with the woman. Her suggestions, however, are based on inferences because she is Emotionally suggestible. It is this difference in suggestibility that necessitates individual sessions with the partners. During the inductions and sessions with the woman, you should slowly increase the number of literal suggestions in each session, a process that aims at creating balanced suggestibility.

As both partners begin to respond well to both literal and inferred suggestions, they may be seen together in therapy, in order to continue strengthening their new communication skills. One means of approaching this is to have them communicate about issues and areas that, in the past, were sources of conflict. Their personal lives, their sexual relationship, financial problems, disputes over in-laws and friends, and other sources of resentment and anger, may be explored. These sessions are aimed at helping both of them take the responsibility to understand each other. The greatest improvements in communication will be witnessed here, as each partner demonstrates an understanding of what the other is saying. The Emotionally suggestible woman, for example, will begin to demonstrate an understanding that, in the past, her partner took most of her communications very literally, when, in fact, she wanted him to infer something else.

The issue of responsibility for communication becomes a two-phased process because each partner must learn to:

1. Take responsibility for making certain he is clearly understood.
2. Take responsibility for understanding his partner.

Each partner should be instructed to practice these responsibilities in therapy sessions by asking after communicating a message, "What did I mean by that?" It is your place, as therapist, to mediate this process by tuning into both the verbal and non-verbal components of messages sent and received by each partner. If the receiver of a message, for instance, turns away and frowns or rolls his eyes up, you may point out that his reaction may indicate that he is denying or ignoring his partner to a certain extent. Your intervention serves to make the receiver consciously aware that he or she must be as open and accepting as possible of his or her partner's communication. The success of the relationship depends on a repeated and successful effort to understand one's partner and to make oneself understood. Success will produce deep sharing and intimacy.

## RELATIONSHIP COUNSELING CASE HISTORY

When a 28-year-old woman came to me for a first consultation, I asked her what had brought her in. She related that she was having difficulty in her marriage and that she was sexually unresponsive. It was extremely difficult for her to communicate her feelings to her husband, and every time she tried, they had a violent argument which ended with him calling her "a cold fish who was sick."

I asked her to tell me about her husband's behavior sexually and emotionally and about the duration and course of their relationship. She stated that they met at the beach when she was twenty-five years old and that they were attracted to each other almost instantly. She had just gotten over a relationship with a man who was very possessive and demonstrative and overly sexual. Her problems with him were the same as those she was now having with her husband.

She described him as being very extroverted and very possessive and domineering. He wanted sex every night, and he had even attempted to have her join a sex swap group, where eight couples swapped partners at get-togethers. She refused violently each time he suggested this.

At the beginning of the marriage, she had enjoyed sex as much as he did, but this lasted for only six months, at which time she gradually became less interested in sex. Even though she had never had an orgasm in the so-called *missionary position*, she felt somewhat satisfied through clitoral stimulation. When she expressed sexual disinterest, her husband became angry and accused her of having an affair. Their communication broke off rapidly, and she began to stay up late at night to avoid sex or any other contact with her husband. He began threatening to leave her, but would become very emotionally upset if she agreed to this. At such times, he begged her to try to make the marriage work.

She told me that she would like it to work, if she could feel the same way she did the first six months of the marriage, but she did not know whether her husband would also come into therapy because he did not believe that there was anything wrong with him. I explained to her that I would definitely prefer to see both of them, but each separately at first, and then, later on, together. She agreed to talk to him about it.

I explained Emotional and Physical suggestibility and sexuality to her, and asked her to answer both the suggestibility and sexuality questionnaires for herself and, in addition, to answer the male sexuality questionnaire for her husband, as she thought he would respond. She scored high on the Emotional scale on both tests, and saw her husband as being highly Physically sexual. (See sexuality questionnaires below.)

The following day, I saw her husband. When I asked what I could do for him, he replied, "There's nothing wrong with me. My wife has the problem. Our marriage is in jeopardy, and if she doesn't straighten out, I will leave her."

I explained briefly the Emotionally sexual female, and had him read description of, both, the Emotional female and the Physical male. He agreed that the Emotional female paper described his wife accurately, but said that the Physical male was only partially him. (This is very typical of the Physically sexual male, who does not see himself as others see him.) As a starting point from which to direct the session, I outlined his options for him: One was to make the marriage work; another was to separate, and the last was divorce. He immediately chose to make the marriage work. He also admitted to denigrating his wife during the marriage and to suggesting partner swapping. He claimed that the latter was only to prove to himself that she was not cheating on him because he could not understand why she had become sexually unresponsive.

I suggested that he also take the suggestibility and sexuality questionnaires, in the same way his wife had, and I told him that I would see them both together at the next session. As expected, his scores indicated a high degree of Physical suggestibility and sexuality, and he saw his wife as being Emotionally sexual. (See sexuality questionnaires below.)

The next session was a conjoint session. We first discussed the tests and examined the differences in the ways they saw themselves and each other. We also discussed how the husband had less understanding of his wife's behavior that she had of his. She saw herself as 81% Emotionally sexual; he saw her as 61% Emotionally sexual (twenty points difference). He saw himself as 84% Physically sexual and she saw him as 76% Physically sexual (eight points difference). This indicated that he saw her as more like he wanted her to be than like she really was; and he treated her according to this wishful, but false, perception. This implied to her that he was not accepting her for herself and that he wanted her to change. This started the burning of hostility within her, and coal was added to the fire, when he suggested that they swap partners. She felt that he wanted her only in order to have another woman. When he fell apart emotionally, she lost respect for him because she felt he was weak.

He, in turn, could not understand why she became unresponsive sexually and emotionally, so he pushed her even harder to have more sex, hoping to make it better. This drove them even further apart, and communication continued to diminish, until they arrived at the point where both were so frustrated because they could not understand or be understood, that they wanted to run from the whole situation.

I explained their behavior to both of them, emphasizing that there was no right or wrong to their suggestible or sexual behavior, just that it was exaggerated because of misunderstanding that led to frustration. I assured them that we would take steps to correct this misunderstanding, by learning to communicate properly. The first step in learning effective communication is to judge one's partner only by the partner's behavior, and to avoid making value judgments about rights or wrongs, past relationships, and third parties (such as family and friends). The second step is to take full responsibility for making absolutely sure that what one says is totally understood by one's partner; and the partner being communicated with must take responsibility for understanding what the speaker is saying.

Using the sexuality questionnaires that they had prepared, I read each question on the female questionnaire aloud and asked the wife what she meant by her answers. I then asked the husband to explain how he interpreted her answers. I did the same with the male questionnaire. My purpose was to search out the verbal and extraverbal conflicts. As I saw a conflict, I brought it out and explained it, I continued this process for the next two sessions, and then suggested that I see them individually for a few sessions. During the individual sessions, I used hypnotherapy to desensitize some hostilities that were still present and that were preventing full communication on both sides, and sexual comfort on the wife's part.

During my first session with the wife, I told her what she could expect to feel and experience in the hypnotic state. I then started with an arm-raising test, using literal suggestions, in order to test the results of her written questionnaires. When she failed to respond, I switched over to inferred suggestions. Once the arm reached her forehead, I suggested deep sleep, added a post-hypnotic suggestion to re-hypnosis, and had her open her eyes, while she moved into a recliner chair. There, I had her close her eyes, and I used a progressive relaxation, in order to deepen her state. I also used some physical, literal suggestions involving ego sensations, in an effort to increase her Physical suggestibility.

Once I felt that she was in a state equal to her suggestible potential, I had her go back over different situations involving frustration with her husband, suggesting that she would first feel the frustration and then pass it and feel more relaxed. I then suggested that she attempt to feel a specific frustration again, but added that she would find herself becoming indifferent to it. I continued this process for the next five sessions, until I arrived at the time when I considered it appropriate to work with her desire to participate sexually with her husband. I had her go back in time to the beginning of their relationship, and had her visualize how comfortable she was with him sexually. Then I suggested that she bring that feeling forward to the present time.

At the same time that I was working with the wife, I was also working with her husband and altering his suggestibility more toward a balanced state. To remove his over-possessiveness, I had to remove the feelings of rejection and loss that he felt. I did this by desensitization through visualization and literal suggestions, having him see his wife the way she was during the early part of their relationship.

After a series of hypnotic sessions individually and about four more conjoint sessions, their relationship took an upward turn. They started to share feelings and direction, and planned goals together. This new balance in the relationship emerged after about six months of relationship counseling.

Some time after the relationship counseling was over, I had an appointment with the wife, in which we worked to end her smoking habit. She related to me that their communication is still improving and that their marriage is happier than it has ever been.

## Answers to Sexuality Questionnaire as She Sees Herself (81% Emotional/19% Physical)

# PART ONE

1.In this question, we will use the term "Father" to designate the male parent, step-parent, relative, or other primary role model – the male figure who had the most influence upon you and your life; and we will use the term "Mother" to designate the female parent, step-parent, relative, or other primary role model – the female figure who had the most influence upon you and your life. If more than one of the answers apply, check "Yes" for both. You should answer "Yes," if your father exhibited one or more of the behaviors listed.

a. When you were between the ages of 9 and 14, was your father more possessive of you and/or more physically and verbally expressive of affection for you than your mother was?    Yes (**No**)

b. When you were between the ages of 9 and 14, were you raised by your mother only?

c When you were between the ages of 9 and 14, were you raised by your father only?

2. If your partner ends a relationship that you wish to continue, do you find your thoughts drifting back to your partner and your energies turning toward restoring the relationship, to the point where you find it difficult to concentrate on other things?    Yes (**No**)

3. Is your relationship the "Number 1 Priority" in your life?    (**Yes**) No

4. Do you enjoy selecting and giving gifts to your partner?    Yes (**No**)

5. Do you feel that you demonstrate more outward affection and love toward your partner than he/she does toward you?    (**Yes**) No

6. Are you comfortable when your partner shows you attention or flatters you when others are present?    Yes (**No**)

7. If you suspected your partner of cheating on you, would you lay more blame on the third party who led him/her astray than you would on your partner for being led astray?    Yes (**No**)

8. Is it easier for you to express intimate feelings and attitudes than it is for your partner to do so?    Yes (**No**)

9. Would you find it easy to accept your partner's children from a previous marriage or relationship?    (**Yes**) No

10. Are you more jealous and/or possessive of your partner than he/she is of you?    (**Yes**) No

11. When you and your partner are having sex, do you desire to prolong the act as long as possible or to repeat the act immediately or following a short rest?    Yes (**No**)

12. Would you like your partner to approach you sexually more than he/she does at present?    Yes (**No**)

13. Looking back to a previous relationship, were you ever rejected so badly that you experienced tremendous physical and/or emotional pain as a result?    Yes (**No**)

14. In a past relationship, where you felt you had been rejected, were you capable of extreme anger, tantrums, vindictive behavior toward your partner, or violence? (Answer "Yes," if you felt capable of one or more of these behaviors.)    Yes (**No**)

15. When you first meet a person to whom you are sexually attracted, is your attention initially drawn to the area of the body below the waist, rather than above the waist?    Yes (**No**)

16. Are you more socially outgoing and extroverted than your partner?    Yes (**No**)

17. When there is a problem in your relationship, do you feel that, rather than just letting things "blow over," you need to "talk it out" with your partner before you can again feel secure in the relationship?               Yes (No)

18. In a relationship, do you have a need for your partner to tell you "where you stand" with him/her?               Yes (No)

19. Do you want to have sex more often than your partner does?               Yes (No)

20. Would you like your partner to talk about what he/she is feeling and experiencing while you are making love.               Yes (No)

## PART TWO

1. In this question, we will use the term "Father" to designate the male parent, step-parent, relative, or other primary role model (the male figure who had the most influence on you and your life) and the term "Mother" to designate the female parent, step-parent, relative, or other primary role model (the female figure who had the most influence on you and your life). If more than one of the answers apply, check "Yes" for both. You should answer "Yes," if your father exhibited one or more of the behaviors listed.

a. When you were between the ages of 9 and 14, was your father less possessive of you and/or less physically and verbally expressive of affection for you than your mother was?               (Yes) No

b. When you were between the ages of 9 and 14, were you raised by your mother only?               Yes No

c. When you were between the ages of 9 and 14, were you raised by your father only?               Yes No

2. Does your anticipation of the pleasure you will receive from sex often exceed the pleasure you               (Yes) No

actually experience from the act itself?

3. During sex with your partner, do you often fantasize about a different partner or sexual act, in order to become or remain sexually aroused?  Yes (No)

4. Do you often find yourself wanting to hurry up and end the sex act before your partner does?  (Yes) No

5. During sex with your partner, is it more of a turn-off than a turn-on, if our partner kisses you heavily?  (Yes) No

6. During a single evening or session of lovemaking, after you and your partner have had sex, does he/she usually want to have sex again before you do?  (Yes) No

7. Shortly after you complete the sexual act, do you feel a desire to fall asleep, move away from your partner, or to engage in some non-sexual activity (reading, watching television, taking a shower, etc.), rather than "cuddle" with your partner? (Answer "Yes," if you feel the desire, whether or not you actually do engage in the other activity.)  (Yes) No

8. After the newness of a relationship wears off, do you find that your sex drive diminishes to a level where it is appreciably lower than your partner's?  (Yes) No

9. Thinking back to the end of a previous relationship, did you already have a new partner in mind, or were you already involved with someone else before the relationship ended?  (Yes) No

10. If your partner talks about the sex act while you are having intercourse, do you find it harder to concentrate on your sexual feelings?  (Yes) No

11. Do you feel comfortable, if your partner touches, kisses, or handles you in public?  (Yes) No

12. Do you find excuses not to have sex with your partner more often than your partner makes excuses  Yes (No)

not to have sex with you?

13. After you and your partner have resolved an argument or disagreement, does it usually take you a longer time than your partner to "forgive and forget" and get back into the mood to have sex with him/her? **(Yes)** No

14. Does it bother or annoy you to have to give your partner frequent reassurance and compliments? **(Yes)** No

15. Do you seem to need more "alone time" away from your partner than he or she needs away from you? **(Yes)** No

16. Instead of talking about your relationship, do you usually take the attitude that, as long as you don't complain, everything is okay? **(Yes)** No

17. When you and your partner are making love, does it make you uncomfortable, if your partner talks explicitly about what he or she is feeling or doing, or asks you to talk about what you are feeling or doing? **(Yes)** No

18. When you first meet a person to whom you are sexually attracted, is your attention initially drawn to the area of the body above the waist, rather from the waist down? **(Yes)** No

19. Do you think you are capable of being in love with more than one person at the same time? Yes (No) Yes **(No)**

20. Does your partner want sex more often than you do? **(Yes)** No

## Answers to Sexuality Questionnaire as He Sees Her (61% Emotional/39% Physical)

## PART ONE

1. In this question, we will use the term "Father" to designate the male parent, step-parent, relative, or other primary role model – the male figure who had the most influence upon you and your life; and we will use the term "Mother" to designate the female parent,

step-parent, relative, or other primary role model – the female figure who had the most influence upon you and your life. If more than one of the answers apply, check "Yes" for both. You should answer "Yes," if your father exhibited one or more of the behaviors listed.

a. When you were between the ages of 9 and 14, was your father more possessive of you and/or more physically and verbally expressive of affection for you than your mother was?　　Yes **No**

b. When you were between the ages of 9 and 14, were you raised by your mother only?　　Yes No

c. When you were between the ages of 9 and 14, were you raised by your father only?　　Yes No

2. If your partner ends a relationship that you wish to continue, do you find your thoughts drifting back to your partner and your energies turning toward restoring the relationship, to the point where you find it difficult to concentrate on other things?　　Yes **No**

3. Is your relationship the "Number 1 Priority" in your life?　　**Yes** No

4. Do you enjoy selecting and giving gifts to your partner?　　Yes **No**

5. Do you feel that you demonstrate more outward affection and love toward your partner than he/she does toward you?　　**Yes** No

6. Are you comfortable when your partner shows you attention or flatters you when others are present?　　**Yes** No

7. If you suspected your partner of cheating on you, would you lay more blame on the third party who led him/her astray than you would on your partner for being led astray?　　Yes **No**

8. Is it easier for you to express intimate feelings and attitudes than it is for your partner to do so?　　Yes **No**

9. Would you find it easy to accept your partner's children from a previous marriage or relationship? **(Yes)** No

10. Are you more jealous and/or possessive of your partner than he/she is of you? **(Yes)** No

11. When you and your partner are having sex, do you desire to prolong the act as long as possible or to repeat the act immediately or following a short rest? Yes **(No)**

12. Would you like your partner to approach you sexually more than he/she does at present? Yes **(No)**

13. Looking back to a previous relationship, were you ever rejected so badly that you experienced tremendous physical and/or emotional pain as a result? Yes **(No)**

14. In a past relationship, where you felt you had been rejected, were you capable of extreme anger, tantrums, vindictive behavior toward your partner, or violence? (Answer "Yes," if you felt capable of one or more of these behaviors.) **(Yes)** No

15. When you first meet a person to whom you are sexually attracted, is your attention initially drawn to the area of the body below the waist, rather than above the waist? Yes **(No)**

16. Are you more socially outgoing and extroverted than your partner? Yes **(No)**

17. When there is a problem in your relationship, do you feel that, rather than just letting things "blow over," you need to "talk it out" with your partner before you can again feel secure in the relationship? Yes **(No)**

18. In a relationship, do you have a need for your partner to tell you "where you stand" with him/her? **(Yes)** No

19. Do you want to have sex more often than your partner does? Yes **(No)**

20. Would you like your partner to talk about what he/she is feeling and experiencing while you are making love. Yes (No)                    Yes (No)

## PART TWO

1. In this question, we will use the term "Father" to designate the male parent, step-parent, relative, or other primary role model (the male figure who had the most influence on you and your life) and the term "Mother" to designate the female parent, step-parent, relative, or other primary role model (the female figure who had the most influence on you and your life). If more than one of the answers apply, check "Yes" for both. You should answer "Yes," if your father exhibited one or more of the behaviors listed.

a. When you were between the ages of 9 and 14, was your father less possessive of you and/or less physically and verbally expressive of affection for you than your mother was?          (Yes) No

b. When you were between the ages of 9 and 14, were you raised by your mother only?          Yes No

c. When you were between the ages of 9 and 14, were you raised by your father only?          Yes No

2. Does your anticipation of the pleasure you will receive from sex often exceed the pleasure you actually experience from the act itself?          Yes (No)

3. During sex with your partner, do you often fantasize about a different partner or sexual act, in order to become or remain sexually aroused?          Yes (No)

4. Do you often find yourself wanting to hurry up and end the sex act before your partner does?          Yes (No)

5. During sex with your partner, is it more of a turn-off than a turn-on, if our partner kisses you heavily?          (Yes) No

6. During a single evening or session of lovemaking, after you and your partner have had sex, does he/she usually want to have sex again before you do?  Yes (No)

7. Shortly after you complete the sexual act, do you feel a desire to fall asleep, move away from your partner, or to engage in some non-sexual activity (reading, watching television, taking a shower, etc.), rather than "cuddle" with your partner? (Answer "Yes," if you feel the desire, whether or not you actually do engage in the other activity.)  Yes (No)

8. After the newness of a relationship wears off, do you find that your sex drive diminishes to a level where it is appreciably lower than your partner's?  (Yes) No

9. Thinking back to the end of a previous relationship, did you already have a new partner in mind, or were you already involved with someone else before the relationship ended?  Yes (No)

10. If your partner talks about the sex act while you are having intercourse, do you find it harder to concentrate on your sexual feelings?  (Yes) No

11. Do you feel comfortable, if your partner touches, kisses, or handles you in public?  Yes (No)

12. Do you find excuses not to have sex with your partner more often than your partner makes excuses not to have sex with you?  (Yes) No

13. After you and your partner have resolved an argument or disagreement, does it usually take you a longer time than your partner to "forgive and forget" and get back into the mood to have sex with him/her?  (Yes) No

14. Does it bother or annoy you to have to give your partner frequent reassurance and compliments?  Yes (No)

15. Do you seem to need more "alone time" away from  Yes (No)

your partner than he or she needs away from you?

16. Instead of talking about your relationship, do you usually take the attitude that, as long as you don't complain, everything is okay?  **(Yes)** No

17. When you and your partner are making love, does it make you uncomfortable, if your partner talks explicitly about what he or she is feeling or doing, or asks you to talk about what you are feeling or doing?  **(Yes)** No

18. When you first meet a person to whom you are sexually attracted, is your attention initially drawn to the area of the body above the waist, rather from the waist down?  Yes **(No)**

19. Do you think you are capable of being in love with more than one person at the same time?  Yes **(No)**

20. Does your partner want sex more often than you do?  **(Yes)** No

## Answers to Sexuality Questionnaire as He Sees Himself (16% Emotional/84% Physical)

1. In this question, we will use the term "Father" to designate the male parent, step-parent, relative, or other primary role model – the male figure who had the most influence upon you and your life; and we will use the term "Mother" to designate the female parent, step-parent, relative, or other primary role model – the female figure who had the most influence upon you and your life. If more than one of the answers apply, check "Yes" for both. You should answer "Yes," if your father exhibited one or more of the behaviors listed.

a. When you were between the ages of 9 and 14, was your father more possessive of you and/or more physically and verbally expressive of affection for you than your mother was?  **(Yes)** No

b. When you were between the ages of 9 and 14, were  Yes No

you raised by your mother only?

c. When you were between the ages of 9 and 14, were you raised by your father only?   Yes  No

2. If your partner ends a relationship that you wish to continue, do you find your thoughts drifting back to your partner and your energies turning toward restoring the relationship, to the point where you find it difficult to concentrate on other things?   **Yes**  No

3. Is your relationship the "Number 1 Priority" in your life?   **Yes**  No

4. Do you enjoy selecting and giving gifts to your partner?   **Yes**  No

5. Do you feel that you demonstrate more outward affection and love toward your partner than he/she does toward you?   Yes  **No**

6. Are you comfortable when your partner shows you attention or flatters you when others are present?   **Yes**  No

7. If you suspected your partner of cheating on you, would you lay more blame on the third party who led him/her astray than you would on your partner for being led astray?   Yes  **No**

8. Is it easier for you to express intimate feelings and attitudes than it is for your partner to do so?   **Yes**  No

9. Would you find it easy to accept your partner's children from a previous marriage or relationship?   **Yes**  No

10. Are you more jealous and/or possessive of your partner than he/she is of you?   **Yes**  No

11. When you and your partner are having sex, do you desire to prolong the act as long as possible or to repeat the act immediately or following a short rest?   **Yes**  No

12. Would you like your partner to approach you   **Yes**  No

sexually more than he/she does at present?

13. Looking back to a previous relationship, were you ever rejected so badly that you experienced tremendous physical and/or emotional pain as a result? **(Yes)** No

14. In a past relationship, where you felt you had been rejected, were you capable of extreme anger, tantrums, vindictive behavior toward your partner, or violence? (Answer "Yes," if you felt capable of one or more of these behaviors.) Yes **(No)**

15. When you first meet a person to whom you are sexually attracted, is your attention initially drawn to the area of the body below the waist, rather than above the waist? **(Yes)** No

16. Are you more socially outgoing and extroverted than your partner? **(Yes)** No

17. When there is a problem in your relationship, do you feel that, rather than just letting things "blow over," you need to "talk it out" with your partner before you can again feel secure in the relationship? Yes **(No)**

18. In a relationship, do you have a need for your partner to tell you "where you stand" with him/her? **(Yes)** No

19. Do you want to have sex more often than your partner does? **(Yes)** No

20. Would you like your partner to talk about what he/she is feeling and experiencing while you are making love. **(Yes)** No

## PART TWO

1. In this question, we will use the term "Father" to designate the male parent, step-parent, relative, or other primary role model (the male figure who had the most influence on you and your life) and the term "Mother" to designate the female parent, step-parent,

relative, or other primary role model (the female figure who had the most influence on you and your life). If more than one of the answers apply, check "Yes" for both. You should answer "Yes," if your father exhibited one or more of the behaviors listed.

a. When you were between the ages of 9 and 14, was your father less possessive of you and/or less physically and verbally expressive of affection for you than your mother was?    Yes (No)

b. When you were between the ages of 9 and 14, were you raised by your mother only?    Yes No

c. When you were between the ages of 9 and 14, were you raised by your father only?    Yes No

2. Does your anticipation of the pleasure you will receive from sex often exceed the pleasure you actually experience from the act itself?    Yes (No)

3. During sex with your partner, do you often fantasize about a different partner or sexual act, in order to become or remain sexually aroused?    (Yes) No

4. Do you often find yourself wanting to hurry up and end the sex act before your partner does?    Yes (No)

5. During sex with your partner, is it more of a turn-off than a turn-on, if our partner kisses you heavily?    Yes (No)

6. During a single evening or session of lovemaking, after you and your partner have had sex, does he/she usually want to have sex again before you do?    Yes (No)

7. Shortly after you complete the sexual act, do you feel a desire to fall asleep, move away from your partner, or to engage in some non-sexual activity (reading, watching television, taking a shower, etc.), rather than "cuddle" with your partner? (Answer "Yes," if you feel the desire, whether or not you    Yes (No)

actually do engage in the other activity.)

8. After the newness of a relationship wears off, do you find that your sex drive diminishes to a level where it is appreciably lower than your partner's?    Yes (No)

9. Thinking back to the end of a previous relationship, did you already have a new partner in mind, or were you already involved with someone else before the relationship ended?    Yes (No)

10. If your partner talks about the sex act while you are having intercourse, do you find it harder to concentrate on your sexual feelings?    Yes (No)

11. Do you feel comfortable, if your partner touches, kisses, or handles you in public?    Yes (No)

12. Do you find excuses not to have sex with your partner more often than your partner makes excuses not to have sex with you?    Yes (No)

13. After you and your partner have resolved an argument or disagreement, does it usually take you a longer time than your partner to "forgive and forget" and get back into the mood to have sex with him/her?    Yes (No)

14. Does it bother or annoy you to have to give your partner frequent reassurance and compliments?    Yes (No)

15. Do you seem to need more "alone time" away from your partner than he or she needs away from you?    Yes (No)

16. Instead of talking about your relationship, do you usually take the attitude that, as long as you don't complain, everything is okay?    (Yes) No

17. When you and your partner are making love, does it make you uncomfortable, if your partner talks explicitly about what he or she is feeling or doing, or asks you to talk about what you are feeling or doing?    Yes (No)

18. When you first meet a person to whom you are sexually attracted, is your attention initially drawn to the area of the body above the waist, rather from the waist down?     Yes **(No)**

19. Do you think you are capable of being in love with more than one person at the same time?     **(Yes)** No

20. Does your partner want sex more often than you do?     Yes **(No)**

## Answers to Sexuality Questionnaire as She Sees Him (76% Physical/24% Emotional)

## PART ONE

1. In this question, we will use the term "Father" to designate the male parent, step-parent, relative, or other primary role model – the male figure who had the most influence upon you and your life; and we will use the term "Mother" to designate the female parent, step-parent, relative, or other primary role model – the female figure who had the most influence upon you and your life. If more than one of the answers apply, check "Yes" for both. You should answer "Yes," if your father exhibited one or more of the behaviors listed.

a. When you were between the ages of 9 and 14, was your father more possessive of you and/or more physically and verbally expressive of affection for you than your mother was?     **(Yes)** No

b. When you were between the ages of 9 and 14, were you raised by your mother only?     Yes No

c. When you were between the ages of 9 and 14, were you raised by your father only?     Yes No

2. If your partner ends a relationship that you wish to continue, do you find your thoughts drifting back to your partner and your energies turning toward restoring the relationship, to the point where you find     **(Yes)** No

it difficult to concentrate on other things?

3. Is your relationship the "Number 1 Priority" in your life?  Yes (No)

4. Do you enjoy selecting and giving gifts to your partner?  Yes (No)

5. Do you feel that you demonstrate more outward affection and love toward your partner than he/she does toward you?  Yes (No)

6. Are you comfortable when your partner shows you attention or flatters you when others are present?  (Yes) No

7. If you suspected your partner of cheating on you, would you lay more blame on the third party who led him/her astray than you would on your partner for being led astray?  Yes (No)

8. Is it easier for you to express intimate feelings and attitudes than it is for your partner to do so?  (Yes) No

9. Would you find it easy to accept your partner's children from a previous marriage or relationship?  (Yes) No

10. Are you more jealous and/or possessive of your partner than he/she is of you?  (Yes) No

11. When you and your partner are having sex, do you desire to prolong the act as long as possible or to repeat the act immediately or following a short rest?  Yes (No)

12. Would you like your partner to approach you sexually more than he/she does at present?  (Yes) No

13. Looking back to a previous relationship, were you ever rejected so badly that you experienced tremendous physical and/or emotional pain as a result?  (Yes) No

14. In a past relationship, where you felt you had been rejected, were you capable of extreme anger, tantrums, vindictive behavior toward your partner, or violence?  Yes (No)

(Answer "Yes," if you felt capable of one or more of these behaviors.)

15. When you first meet a person to whom you are sexually attracted, is your attention initially drawn to the area of the body below the waist, rather than above the waist?  **[Yes]** No

16. Are you more socially outgoing and extroverted than your partner?  **[Yes]** No

17. When there is a problem in your relationship, do you feel that, rather than just letting things "blow over," you need to "talk it out" with your partner before you can again feel secure in the relationship?  Yes **[No]**

18. In a relationship, do you have a need for your partner to tell you "where you stand" with him/her?  **[Yes]** No

19. Do you want to have sex more often than your partner does?  **[Yes]** No

20. Would you like your partner to talk about what he/she is feeling and experiencing while you are making love.  Yes **[No]**

## PART TWO

1. In this question, we will use the term "Father" to designate the male parent, step-parent, relative, or other primary role model (the male figure who had the most influence on you and your life) and the term "Mother" to designate the female parent, step-parent, relative, or other primary role model (the female figure who had the most influence on you and your life). If more than one of the answers apply, check "Yes" for both. You should answer "Yes," if your father exhibited one or more of the behaviors listed.

a. When you were between the ages of 9 and 14, was your father less possessive of you and/or less  Yes **[No]** physically and verbally expressive of affection for you than your mother?

b. When you were between the ages of 9 and 14, were you raised by your mother only? Yes No

c. When you were between the ages of 9 and 14, were you raised by your father only? Yes No

2. Does your anticipation of the pleasure you will receive from sex often exceed the pleasure you actually experience from the act itself? Yes **No**

3. During sex with your partner, do you often fantasize about a different partner or sexual act, in order to become or remain sexually aroused? Yes **No**

4. Do you often find yourself wanting to hurry up and end the sex act before your partner does? Yes **No**

5. During sex with your partner, is it more of a turn-off than a turn-on, if our partner kisses you heavily? Yes **No**

6. During a single evening or session of lovemaking, after you and your partner have had sex, does he/she usually want to have sex again before you do? Yes **No**

7. Shortly after you complete the sexual act, do you feel a desire to fall asleep, move away from your partner, or to engage in some non-sexual activity (reading, watching television, taking a shower, etc.), rather than "cuddle" with your partner? (Answer "Yes," if you feel the desire, whether or not you actually do engage in the other activity.) Yes **No**

8. After the newness of a relationship wears off, do you find that your sex drive diminishes to a level where it is appreciably lower than your partner's? Yes **No**

9. Thinking back to the end of a previous relationship, did you already have a new partner in mind, or were you already involved with someone else before the

relationship ended?

10. If your partner talks about the sex act while you are having intercourse, do you find it harder to concentrate on your sexual feelings? **(Yes)** No

11. Do you feel comfortable, if your partner touches, kisses, or handles you in public? Yes **(No)**

12. Do you find excuses not to have sex with your partner more often than your partner makes excuses not to have sex with you? Yes **(No)**

13. After you and your partner have resolved an argument or disagreement, does it usually take you a longer time than your partner to "forgive and forget" and get back into the mood to have sex with him/her? **(Yes)** No

14. Does it bother or annoy you to have to give your partner frequent reassurance and compliments? Yes **(No)**

15. Do you seem to need more "alone time" away from your partner than he or she needs away from you? Yes **(No)**

16. Instead of talking about your relationship, do you usually take the attitude that, as long as you don't complain, everything is okay? **(Yes)** No

17. When you and your partner are making love, does it make you uncomfortable, if your partner talks explicitly about what he or she is feeling or doing, or asks you to talk about what you are feeling or doing? Yes **(No)**

18. When you first meet a person to whom you are sexually attracted, is your attention initially drawn to the area of the body above the waist, rather from the waist down? Yes **(No)**

19. Do you think you are capable of being in love with more than one person at the same time? **(Yes)** No

20. Does your partner want sex more often than you do? Yes **(No)**

# ADDENDUM TO CASE HISTORY

The case history of the Emotional female and Physical male was selected because it depicts the majority of couples who enter counseling with troubled relationships. Although the opposite situation (in which the male is Emotional and the female is Physical) has been covered at length in this chapter and in Chapter Five, I feel that a brief summary of the major problem areas that characterize such relationships will help you to formulate a distinct and lasting mental picture of each so that you will be able to almost immediately distinguish which of the two situations you are encountering, when someone seeks your help for relationship counseling.

With the Emotional male and Physical female, problems usually begin once the newness of the relationship wears off, at which time the Emotional male begins to withdraw into himself more. At this time, he tends to put more energy into his work than into his home life or sex with his wife. With his wife, he is primarily interested in his own sexual gratification. He also may try to recapture the romance of an early relationship, by keeping one or several mistresses. This kind of behavior, even before it becomes extreme, elicits tremendous feelings of rejection in his Physical wife, and these feelings of rejection compound her naturally jealous, suspicious, and possessive sexual nature. She tries to bring the relationship into balance her way, but because she judges her partner as she judges herself, they are in constant conflict. The more she wants, the less he wants. He feels pressured and withdraws; she feels rejected and pushes more.

In a situation like this, it is imperative that both partners be willing to enter counseling. Unfortunately, the Emotional male seldom will readily agree to conjoint counseling, since he insists that marital problems are the fault of his wife. It is terribly important that he be available for therapy, so a phone call to motivate him may be necessary. In this case, tell him that his constant search for romance and excitement is futile and that if he continues without help, he will spend his life in a continual futile search, drained by alimony, child support, and legal fees. This should motivate him.

Once both partners are in counseling, give them a non-threatening label of suggestibility and a non-punitive explanation of their behavior. Then help the Physical wife feel secure in her womanhood so that her Emotional husband's distance will no longer be such a threat to her. Also, teach her (and her husband) how to judge each other by the other's standards. Work with the Emotional male, by helping him to understand his own behavior and his earlier misunderstandings of it. This should eliminate his restless searching, and this (in combination with his wife's new security and understanding) will establish the relationship on a much more secure footing.

## ADVANTAGES OF HYPNOTIC INTERVENTION IN RELATIONSHIP COUNSELING

The approach to relationship counseling discussed in this chapter, as it applies to both heterosexual and homosexual couples, has a number of advantages over other methods. One of these advantages is that it directs the attention of each partner to the way in which he communicates and the way in which his partner communicates. This leads to efforts that aim toward clarification of communication, a process that is generally seen as necessary for the improvement of marital relations. A second advantage of this approach is that the examination of communication styles and resultant efforts at clarifying communication occurs in what might be referred to as a *no-fault atmosphere*. That is, with each partner understanding that his/her suggestibility type and communication style is normal and acceptable and that his/her partner's suggestibility type and communication style is normal and acceptable as well, therapy may proceed with each partner free from:

1. Blaming his/her partner for all the difficulties experienced in communication.
2. Blaming himself/herself and feeling guilty about being the cause of conflict.

Suggestibility can be described as a trait that is acquired through natural learning processes and, as such, is a quality that no individual consciously controls, as it is being developed.

Consequently, the communication style one acquires is not intentionally developed. Hence, when two individuals arrive at a point in their relationship where their communication styles are a source of conflict, they may be presented with this line of thinking so that neither partner will attempt to attach blame for the conflict on either himself/herself or his/her partner. This is advantageous in that it removes feelings of guilt, hostility, and defensiveness that may create barriers to communication between the partners.

The therapy plan may be viewed from another perspective, in order to shed light on an additional advantage of this approach. You are essentially saying to the couple:

1. You report a problem.
2. My feeling is that neither of you is to be blamed for this problem.
3. Your difficulties lie in an area that is observable in hypnosis, that area being suggestibility.
4. Suggestibility influences your communication with each other.
5. Suggestibility is something that I, as a hypnotist, am able to work with and alter, in order to improve your problematic situation.
6. As I alter your suggestibilities, your communication with each other will improve.

This entire approach is based on the principle that makes hypnosis effective – suggestion. The suggestion is made in the waking state, as well as in hypnotic sessions. The power of suggestion is effective with both partners, if employed as outlined here, in that it literally and inferentially suggests to the couple that they will improve, thereby tapping the receptive areas in both cooperating partners.

Another important advantage in utilizing the terms of Emotional/Physical suggestible and sexual behaviors is that, changing the language to which the couple is accustomed and giving them a new language to learn, starts them on an equal footing, eliminating the *one-up, one-down aspect*. The labels of Emotional and Physical suggestibility are not considered negative because it is explained that these labels are normal for them. Psychological terms, which tend to involve certain amounts of self-fulfilling prophecy, are totally eliminated.

There is one final advantage to be noted. In earlier behavioral approaches, relationship counseling was done with only one partner present. Communication skills could thus not be worked on directly; and the counselor and partner in therapy were often seen by the absent partner as *ganging up* on him. his may actually have occurred, but even if it did not, the absent partner became increasingly reluctant to enter a counseling situation, where he felt that he would be attacked. The hypnotherapeutic model of relationship counseling avoids these problems. A reluctant partner will soon see that the counseling is done in a *no-fault atmosphere*, which will encourage him to come in. With both partners in therapy, their communication can be observed and worked on directly, and both suggestibilities can be changed. If both partners are in counseling, each will know that there are no secret partnerships with the therapist and that there is no *ganging up*. And, finally, the partners will grow and develop (through the counseling situation) *together*.

# CHAPTER 9 – LECTURING AND DEMONSTRATING HYPNOSIS

## GENERAL GUIDELINES

As a hypnotherapist, you are in the unique position of being able to simultaneously lecture about and demonstrate aspects of your profession as a form of ethical advertising. When doing so, it is important that you keep in mind that you are representing a responsible and respectable profession, and that you reflect this attitude in your dress, your personal mannerisms, and your professionalism, as you proceed to establish rapport with the audience.

Always gear your pre-induction speech to the age group and the socio-economic class of the audience, also taking into account why that particular audience would need, or could use, hypnotherapy.

Your subject matter should be directed at informing, not entertaining the public. Avoid the flamboyant, dominant attitude of the stage hypnotist. Even though stage hypnosis has educated the public about some of the uses of hypnosis, it is also responsible for widespread misconceptions about the hypnotic state and about the character of the hypnotist himself.

If you wish to draw subjects from the audience, the best approach is to ask the audience to participate in a hand-clasp, arm-raising, or finger-spreading test. Those who respond most readily to the test can be asked to volunteer as demonstrating subjects. The demonstrations should be in good taste and should never place the subject in an embarrassing or uncontrolled situation. Showing the difference between total tension and total relaxation through an arm-rigidity test, or creating the presence or absence of *stage fright* in front of the group are both tasteful demonstrations.

If you choose to hypnotize the entire audience, follow the procedure of the progressive relaxation induction outlined in Chapter Three. Explain to your audience that this is a basic approach to the first stages of hypnosis and that everyone will enter according to his own suggestibility. Tell them that suggestibility is a learned behavior and that it encompasses how one learns, how one responds to inferences, and how one is affected by the influencing factors of life.

It is possible (and preferable) to maintain total maternalism throughout your presentation, constantly reinforcing the concept that hypnosis is the process of allowing oneself to experience the peaks of receptive suggestibility.

The following is a step-by-step checklist for use in the preparation of a lecture/demonstration on hypnosis:

1. Prepare a pre-induction speech that includes an explanation of the theory of mind; what hypnosis is and is not; and the many and varied uses of hypnosis in today's society.
2. Explain Emotional and Physical suggestibility and how they are created.
3. Discuss hypersuggestibility – what it is, how it is caused, and its dangers.
4. Explain how a person will feel in the hypnotic state, how he will be awakened, and how he will feel following hypnosis.
5. Perform a series of tests on the audience as a whole, or do a progressive relaxation.
6. Perform any additional demonstrations with selected subjects, as desired. Remember to keep this in good taste.
7. Conduct a question-and-answer session, and let people know where you can be reached for consultation. Have business cards and/or brochures available for those who want them.

# CHAPTER 10 – SELF-HYPNOSIS

# MISCONCEPTIONS ABOUT SELF-HYPNOSIS

The basic difference between hetero-hypnosis and self-hypnosis is that hetero-hypnosis involves the disorganization of the inhibitory processes, whereas true self-hypnosis requires the organization of the inhibitory processes. In the hetero-hypnotic state, the hypnotist, by his attitude, technique, and experience, influences his subjects to accept their own suggestibility. Whether it is through inferences, as with the Emotionally suggestible subject, or literally, as with the Physical subject, the operator builds expectation, until he is able to bring about disorganization in the subject's mind and, thereby, create hypersuggestibility.

People are often deluded into believing that they are learning self-hypnosis from hypnotists, who actually use a form of progressive relaxation to hypnotize their clients. The operator will give a post-suggestion to re-hypnosis, which can then be used to make the subject believe that, when he enters the hypnotic state at home, he is entering self-hypnosis. In actuality, however, he is merely responding to the post-hypnotic suggestion. When an individual becomes hypnotized in this manner, he is suggestible only to thoughts and ideas that the hypnotist has given him previously. Anything else that he suggests will not affect him because he is not the one who actually induced the state, and he is suggestible only to the operator who did. Further, after the post-suggestion depreciates (as it will without reinforcement), the subject will no longer be able to enter this so-called *self-hypnotic state*. Individuals who learn this approach usually cease to use self-hypnosis after a short time because they obtain poor results.

Another misconception regarding self-hypnosis should also be cleared up. When you enter the state of self-hypnosis, do not be discouraged when you do not experience ringing bells, flashes of lightning, or feelings of dropping into a bottomless pit. Nothing that occurs is in any way comparable to these dramatic, romantic notions. In most cases, the self-induced hypnotic state is at first, hardly, if at all, recognizable. While in the state, you will hear everything around you, but will feel as if you are in a daydreaming state of relaxation. You may find that your mind wanders, and you may feel numbness or tingling sensations in your fingers or toes or dissociation in part or all of your body. These feelings are natural to self-hypnosis.

Contrary to popular belief, we have found that there is a far greater need for people to be hypnotized than for people to hypnotize themselves. The reason for this is that most individuals who seek help through hypnosis have tried other forms of help to no avail. Usually, they have already tried to deal with their problems on their own and have failed. If a person has such a background of failure, allowing him to hypnotize himself will hardly reverse the trend. Further, in many cases, it is too difficult for a person to be objective about his own problems and, therefore, self-hypnosis will not work for him because he will not know what type of suggestions to give himself. Very depressed individuals will actually take the depression into self-hypnosis with them and may even magnify it, instead of removing it. This type of person tends to think negatively and might create additional problems with negatively worded suggestions.

Based on these facts, you can see that it is not always advisable to teach self-hypnosis to certain people. When you have worked with them privately and helped them to see their problems more objectively, then they will be in a better position to help themselves.

## SELF-HYPNOSIS CONDITIONING

Two Laws of the Mind govern self-hypnosis conditioning; the Law of Repetition and the Law of Association, in that order. The self-hypnosis conditioning process is based on the concept of the three areas of suggestibility (Physical, Emotional, Intellectual). We have found that the human being is directly affected by words and sounds or by the meaning he indirectly infers from them. Since the ideal state in self-hypnosis is achieved when the physical body, the emotions, and the intellect are stimulated, the self-hypnotic state is created with words that will affect all three areas independently. The keywords you select for this purpose will evolve into a personal formula for entering self-hypnosis.

Before you begin the conditioning process, it is important to understand the interrelationship between your emotional and physical responses. Whenever you feel anything emotionally, your body will respond; and any time you feel something physically, your emotions will respond. When one takes place, the other must follow, so a natural association forms between the two. It is a reversible cause and effect relationship – the cause produces the effect, and the effect can reproduce the cause. This concept can be utilized very effectively in your practice sessions.

To practice the conditioning process, first place yourself in a semi-comfortable position. This is more effective than a totally comfortable position because you remain more aware and are, therefore, more able to formulate suggestions and to organize your thought process. Also, a semi-comfortable position prevents you from drifting into a normal sleep state. If you practice self-hypnosis lying down in bed, the natural association of inhibiting the brain and allowing yourself to drift into a normal sleep state will take place. Because this is a stronger condition in the mind than the new condition of hypnotic sleep, it is important that you assume a different position, possibly in a recliner. If you must use your bed, prop yourself up with pillows so that your head is at least twelve inches above your legs. In this position, your mind will not associate with the condition of sleep.

Once you are in a semi-comfortable position, become aware of yourself. Move around until you feel your body floating freely, without restrictions caused by tightness of clothing or any uncomfortable pressure. Let your mind drift over your entire body. This dispatches message units to your brain and prepares you for the condition of fight or flight, which lies very deep in the primitive area of mind. Note, however, that your *fight* reaction will be neutralized by your conscious awareness of what is happening.

In most cases, when a person concentrates on relaxing his body, he either begins with the head area moving downward to the feet or from the feet moving upward to the head. With this new process of conditioning, however, you will begin with your hands, where the greatest skin resistance change takes place, and utilize this awareness of physiological changes taking place in the body.

The first stop in self-hypnosis conditioning is to find the physical stimulus or the word that will create physical changes, known as ego sensations. To do this, lie in a very still position and concentrate on your hands. Just by this simple act of concentration, you will begin to feel some physiological change take place. To demonstrate this to yourself, hold your hand up in front of you and stare at your fingers, attempting to feel some tingling sensation or numbness, as if whatever is inside of the skin is expanding and trying to move outward. Then take your hand and place it back on the chair, continuing to be aware of this feeling. Does your hand feel cold or numb? Is it feeling relaxed? Is it heavy? Is it light? Pick one feeling and one word to which you can relate and try to match the word to the feeling. Concentrate on your hands for approximately three to five minutes; and when you experience the feeling very strongly, say the word to yourself.

For example, you might say to yourself, "I'm feeling a tingling, cold sensation – a cold and tingling sensation." Now take the words cold and tingling and try to recognize which of the two you are feeling more. The one you feel more strongly will become your physical keyword. When you have established your physical key, experiment by laying your hands across the top of your legs, attempting to move the feeling associated with our physical keyword through your thighs and hips, down into calves of your legs and into your feet. While you are practicing, it is always better to remove your shoes so that your feet are exposed to the air around them. This will increase the ego sensations.

Once the physical keyword sensation is achieved and controlled, the Law of Association comes into effect and prepares you for your emotional and intellectual keys. As the physiological change occurs and your mind associates it with your physical keyword, the psychological effect will begin to take place. The fact that you are now feeling or controlling something in your physical body allows your emotions to become active, and leads into your second keyword (your emotional key). At this point, say to yourself:

> *The tingling feeling causes relaxation, moving from my toes to my heels, into my ankles, and into the calves of my legs, and I become aware of my legs pushing down. This tingling sensation is moving back up through my thighs and hips, and I am aware of the contact between my hands and my thighs. This tingling sensation will soon move upward into my arms. As I become aware of my stomach muscles relaxing, I feel this tingling sensation moving upward, and I become aware of my breathing.*

Since your breathing has a stronger effect on emotional change than any other function of your body, it can be utilized to establish and trigger your emotional key. So concentrate on your breathing, until you feel it actually beginning to deepen. Then, become aware of your emotional feelings and attempt to tie in some positive word that will affect your emotional feelings at this particular moment. Since you do not want to associate with any negative emotions, use only positive words, such as *happiness, success, confidence, peacefulness,* or whatever gives you a sensation of elation or well-being. As you say the words, pause between them and become aware of any emotional change that you can feel. If the word is happy, tie in this feeling of happiness with the expansion of your chest and the drawing of new oxygen into your lungs. The word happy will then become your emotional key.

Next, is the intellectual key, which is the third, final and most important in self-hypnosis conditioning. This final key, which is the same for everyone, will be either *deep, hypnotic sleep* or *deep sleep.*

Sleep is a basic need and is the result of a condition to which each of us has been responding since the day we were born. It is a condition we experience every night, when we lie down and place ourselves in a comfortable position, allowing the mind to become inhibited, go almost blank for a few moments, and then drift into the normal escape mechanism of sleep. Your subconscious mind can associate only with a condition, so each time you place yourself in this position, your subconscious mind assumes you are going to sleep, and your conscious mind is allowed to pass into unconsciousness and normal sleep. During this period, the body is allowed to rest, but, more than that, the mind is allowed to vent out through dreams all the events, traumas, thoughts, and ideas that no longer have any value to you. Sleep is a very strong intellectual conditioning. Because you cannot deny the fact that you can, will and must sleep, your intellectual suggestibility (which requires logic and reason) must respond to the suggestion of *deep sleep*.

You can use this condition in self-hypnosis by altering a few aspects of the normal sleep state. First, change the position of the body to eliminate the natural association with normal sleep. Secondly, add *deep hypnotic* or *deep* to the word *sleep* to further distinguish between the two states and to place you in this trance-like state. The fact that you are concentrating on your body, allows you to organize your inhibitory processes. At the beginning, this condition may place you into only a light state, but repetition will bring greater depth and control, and you will form a very strong conditioned response to the three keywords.

Through experimentation, we have found that, in hypnosis, any condition placed properly in the mind approximately twenty-one times becomes an automatic trigger mechanism that continues to grow stronger with use. During the self-hypnosis conditioning process, your eyes may have a tendency to develop rapid-eye movement, identical to that which takes place when you are dreaming, and you may feel your eyes attempting to roll up involuntarily under your eyelids. Utilize this condition by deliberately rolling your eyes up and simultaneously repeating the words, deep hypnotic sleep to yourself, thus developing an association between the eyes rolling up and the words *deep hypnotic sleep*.

Once in the state, you may have a tendency to doubt that you are in hypnosis because of your conscious awareness. However, conscious awareness is actually an indication that you are in the hypnotic state, as opposed to the normal sleep state. Another characteristic of the hypnotic state is that you may, at times, forget what you were concentrating on because, any time your consciousness begins to go into abeyance, it has a tendency to drift from your normal thought process to past events or future plans. You should not attempt to overcome this, but, instead, utilize it in your conditioning process as a very powerful way of expanding your mind and opening it up to the possibility of increasing your psychic awareness. You can further use it to develop positive thoughts and ideas for different types of business transactions, schooling, or whatever.

In summary, the self-hypnosis conditioning procedure is as follows: assuming that your keywords are *tingling, happy,* and *deep hypnotic sleep,* place yourself in a semi-comfortable position, with your hands on your thighs. Begin to concentrate on your hands, suggesting silently to yourself that you feel a tingling sensation in your hands, which begins to move down through your body and into your legs. Once the tingling sensation reaches your feet, reverse the action, suggesting that you feel this tingling sensation from your toes into your heels, your ankles, the calves of your legs, the area where there is contact between your hands and your legs, and then up through your mid-section. As this relaxation begins to move upward through your stomach muscles and solar plexus, become aware that it continues up through your arms. At this time, deepen your breathing and move all your concentration to your breathing, while saying your emotional keyword silently to yourself. This expansion of breathing and the natural association of the word *happy* will begin to represent the condition of your emotional key.

Continue to be aware of your breathing still deepening, as the relaxation moves through your shoulders, into your back, up through your neck muscles, in through your scalp and across your forehead. As it begins to move down over the facial muscles and jaw muscles, become aware that your eyes have a tendency to move upward under your eyelids. As you recognize this physiological movement, implant the words *deep hypnotic sleep* in your mind to strengthen the natural association.

The importance of the next step – the awakening procedure – cannot be emphasized enough. Many times, people who have entered different states of trance will fail to bring themselves out of the state and, so remain very suggestible to themselves and to the negativity in their environment. In fact, many psychologists, psychiatrists, hypnotists, marriage counselors, and other counselors or therapists will find, at one time or another, that they are becoming overly receptive to themselves, as well as to others, for this very reason. If the hypersuggestible condition is not recognized and altered, they may eventually reach a point where they are unable to cope with other people's problems.

The awakening procedure simply consists of establishing a condition that your mind will associate with awakening. The best procedure is to count from zero upward to five and say, "Wide awake!" Then, almost immediately, change your position by sitting up or moving to a different chair or different location. Your mind will perceive this motion as an active, rather than a passive, condition and will, therefore, release you from the hypersuggestible state. Again, repeat the count, "Zero, one, two, three, four, five," and the words, "Wide awake." Just as suggestions reiterated in the mind will create a conditioned response, so the awakening procedure repeated in the mind will create a condition, whereby you are brought back to the waking state.

After you have created both the hypnotic state and the waking state a few times, you will begin to recognize the different feelings associated with each. When entering the hypnotic state, some people will feel a twinge of current pass over their foreheads, some will have a feeling of calmness, some a feeling of numbness, and so on. Each individual will experience his own unique and distinct ego sensation change. Some people feel a slight trembling when they awaken or a difference in alertness, and so forth. It is important that you learn to recognize your own reactions so that you will always be aware of whether you are in or out of the state and will always have full control of your suggestibility.

Because self-hypnosis is a conditioned response, consistent practice is a must. This does not mean that you should spend a great deal of time in the state, but that you should practice often. In fact, fifteen minutes should be the average time spent in the state or the tendency to drift becomes too strong.

Should you be disturbed by the phone ringing or someone coming to the door while you are in hypnosis, be sure to count yourself out. Do not assume that you are out of the state just because your eyes are open and you are walking around. If you neglect to awaken yourself, you will remain suggestible to all the negatives with which you come into contact. Since there are more negatives than positives on the news, in the newspapers, and in everyday life, you will take all of this in, and will probably begin to feel irritable or depressed. If you notice these symptoms and remember that you did not awaken yourself the last time you were in self-hypnosis, simply go through the process of counting yourself in, achieving as great a depth as possible, and then counting yourself out, being sure to say, "Wide awake!"

The degree of success one achieves with self-hypnosis conditioning is determined by the practice time involved. Some can accomplish a self-induced hypersuggestible state in a day, others in a week, while with some, it may take months. But it will work for everyone.

*This page intentionally left blank.*

# GLOSSARY

**ABREACTION** – A physical movement or an emotional outburst as a reaction to a suggestion, while in the state of hypnosis. Some hypnotic abreactions are spontaneous and others are created by the hypnotist. Hypnotic abreaction can be used to acquire greater depth, cause revivification, or remove repressed emotions.

**AFFIRMATIONS** – Positive suggestions given through hypnosis and in Mental Bank ideomotor exercises in order to reprogram one's life script.

**AGE REGRESSION** – The state in which the subject relives past events of his life while in the hypnotic state. If the subject reacts as he did when he was at that younger age, but views the subject matter with his present maturity, it is called *behavioral regression;* if he feels that he is actually at the younger age, it is called *revivification regression.*

**ALPHA** – Slow brainwave activity state of hypnosis (resting but awake). Also known as hypnoidal. Alpha is slower (deeper) than Beta, the awake state, and faster than Theta, a deep hypnotic state.

**AMNESIA** – Loss of memory. The amnesia which frequently occurs in hypnosis may be either spontaneous or induced by suggestion.

**ANCHOR** – A specific stimulus such as a word, image or touch that through the rule of association evokes a particular mental, emotional, and/or physiological state.

**ARM RAISING / PRIMARY INDUCTION** – The Arm Raising Induction is known as the primary induction because it is used only in the first session to create the association of hypnotic depth and establish the expectation of a successful therapy. The therapist is able to use misdirection as well as inferred and literal suggestions in order to affect either the Emotionally or Physically Suggestible client. Through these suggestions, the therapist influences the client's subconscious, causing the arm, from the fingertips to the elbow, to lift up off the table, with the hand eventually making contact with the face. At this point it is stated that they have reached the peak of their suggestibility and a challenge can be given with respect to the client's hand sticking to their face. Deepening techniques would follow.

**ASSOCIATED** – A sub-modality of NLP; a picture or visual image where you see the world out of your own eyes. Contrast with the disassociated state where you visually observe your body from outside the view of your eyes.

**ASSOCIATION** – Also known as Pavlovian conditioning. A process by which a subject comes to respond in a desired manner to a previously neutral stimulus that has been repeatedly presented along with a stimulus that elicits the desired response. Most common Kappasinian association is conditioning the words "deep sleep" with the hypnotic state.

**AUTO DUAL INDUCTION** – An induction primarily given to Intellectual Suggestibles, where the client believes they are hypnotizing themselves. While feeling the pulse in their own outstretched arm, the client repeats what the Hypnotherapist says, leading to a count from five to zero and Deep Sleep.

**AVERSION** – Relating to hearing or sound. One of the three major representational systems of encoding information, alongside visual and kinesthetic.

**BEHAVIOR MODIFICATION** – The process of changing behavior by using techniques based on learning theory. The techniques include systematic desensitization, aversion therapy, and assertion training.

**BELIEFS** – Knowns in the subconscious.

**BETA** – The brainwave activity state of the normal awake state. Higher than Alpha and Theta.

**BODY SYNDROMES** – A body syndrome is a physical manifestation of an emotional trauma. When an emotion is held in or repressed instead of being processed and released, the emotion will express itself as a physical discomfort.

**BUNCHING** – When an individual fails to separate one problem from another or one area of his life from another. In order to help this individual, the operator must help him to separate his problems and handle them individually.

**BUYING THE SYMPTOMS** – Getting a client to accept some of the patterns in their life.

**CATALEPSY** – A medium depth of hypnosis, between *hypnoidal* and *somnambulism*.

**CHAINING ANCHORS** – A Neuro Linguistic (NLP) technique where a group of anchors are fired off one after another. Often used to take a subject from a stuck state to a more resourceful state.

**CHALLENGE** – Essentially a dare in which the hypnotist challenges the client to perform some act which it is impossible for the client to do at his/her depth in the hypnotic state. Examples are the eye challenge and the arm rigidity challenge.

**CHUNKING** – Moving between levels of specificity. To chunk up means to move to the bigger picture, to chunk down would be getting to greater levels of specificity.

**CIRCLE THERAPY** – Use only for the extinction of fears. It is the process of having the client repeatedly confront his problem while in the hypnotic state. Since anxiety and relaxation are incompatible, the anxiety will gradually disappear. After having brought up and passed the fear many times, a reversal is given that the harder he tries to bring up the old fear, the more difficult it becomes. In fact, you will feel a new emotion (replacement), amusement and a tendency to smile.

**CLIMAX** – See *Orgasm*.

**CONDITIONED RESPONSE** – The learned response to an indifferent stimulus, which has been attached to it by repeatedly pairing the stimulus with the reinforcer.

**CONSCIOUS MIND** – The 12% of our mind of which we are most aware. The part responsible for logic, reasoning, decision-making, and will power.

**CONTRADICTORY SQUARE** – An example is when a person with a high IQ is in a job that does not require or will not use the high IQ. The person is in conflict or incongruence between what he IS capable of doing and what he BELIEVES he is capable of doing.

**CONVERSION TO HYPNOSIS** – A suggestibility test (such as the finger-spreading test), which is extended beyond the point where the suggestibility is determined, and is used as an induction into hypnosis (at which point, it is called the *finger-spreading conversion.*)

**CORRECTIVE THERAPY** – The client states their problem in a sentence. Then the client is to list five synonyms to each word in the sentence. Physical Suggestibles keep referring back to the original words in the sentence while Emotional Suggestibles refer to each previous word they've come up with. The last line is the subconscious problem.

**CRITICAL AREA OF MIND** – An area of mind that is part conscious and part subconscious. Any time a suggestion is given to a subject that is detrimental to his well-being or in total opposition to his way of thinking, it will affect critical area of mind, and he will critically reject it by abreacting.

**DEEP SLEEP** – A post-hypnotic suggestion given to a client that capitalizes on the Law of Dominance.

**DEHYPNOTIZATION** – The process of removing a person from a hypersuggestible state.

## DEEPENING TECHNIQUES

**Reactional Hypnosis** – Repeatedly awakening the client and re-hypnotizing him/her with a post-suggestion to re-hypnosis.

**Arm Rigidity** – The Hypnotherapist holds the client's outstretched arm from beneath the elbow. She paternally instructs the client to draw all the tensions of his body into his arm, from the count of five to zero. At zero the arm will be as tight as a steel bar. The client is told the tensions will release, and he'll go deeper when the therapist touches his pulse.

**Heavy Light** – A client's arms are both outstretched, right hand palm up and the left hand at a right angle with thumb up. He is told a weight is placed in his right hand pressing down (literal suggestion) and a powerful helium balloon is tied to his left thumb (inferred suggestion). When right hand touches leg he'll go deeper. A deepening technique and suggestibility test follow.

**Staircase** – Having the client visualize or imagine she is standing at the top of a staircase of twenty steps. The staircase is well lit and has a sturdy handrail. Each step the client imagines herself taking down the staircase will take her deeper into the hypnotic state.

**Eye Fascination** – Client is told to open their eyes and look at the tip of a pen held above client's eye level. They are instructed to follow the pen only with their eyes. As the client's eyes track downward, the lids will close. When they close, the Hypnotherapist touches client's forehead and says "deep sleep."

**Progressive Relaxation** – A deepening technique but also an important secondary induction. The aim of this maternal technique is to relax the various areas of the client's body starting from the feet if he is in the reclined position (from the head down if he is sitting). Once the relaxation is completed toe to head, a five to zero count is given, at which time the Hypnotherapist snaps his/her fingers and says "deep sleep."

**DEFENSE MECHANISMS** – All defense mechanisms stem from the basic instinct of survival. They operate on an unconscious level and they serve to deny or distort reality, thoughts, and action. Some Defense Mechanisms are: Repression, Denial, Rationalization, Projection, Displacement, Turning against self, Reaction Formation, Overcompensation, Intellectualization, Withdrawal, Regression, Sublimation, and Disassociation.

**DELTA** – Slowest brainwave activity pattern of sleep, and the deepest, somnambulistic state of hypnosis. Also see Alpha, Beta and Theta.

## DEPTH

**Hypnoidal** – A light stage of hypnosis, usually associated with emotional suggestibility; also used to refer to the state of consciousness which is passed through in the transition from sleep to waking, and vice versa. It is characterized by rapid eye movement (REM), with an up/down motion of the eyes.

**Cataleptic** – A medium depth of hypnosis. Characterized by a side to side movement of the eyes.

**Somnambulism** – The deepest state of hypnosis, where the client responds with amnesia, anesthesia, negative and positive hallucinations, and complete control of the senses. This type of person usually has 50% emotional suggestibility and 50% physical suggestibility. It is characterized by the eyes rolling up underneath the eyelids.

**DIRECT SUGGESTION** – Hypnotic suggestions in the form of a command or instruction. Contrast to Inferential Suggestion.

**DISSOCIATED** – A sub-modality of NLP; a picture or visual image where you visually observe your body from outside the view of your eyes. Such as seeing your life from the perspective of a camera, or floating above yourself.

**DISSOCIATION** – The loss of feeling in different areas of the body (usually the arms and legs), while in the state of hypnosis; being more aware of mind than of body.

**EGO SENSATION** – Change of feeling in the physical body or part of the body.

**EMOTIONAL AND PHYSICAL SEXUALITY** – The theory of human behavior based upon the idea that an individual's behavior is developed by that person's secondary caretaker. Sexuality is a kind of continuum, with 100% Emotionals or Physicals on either end and the different combinations of the two falling everywhere in the middle.

**EMOTIONAL SEXUALITY** – A type of sexual behavior in which the individual reacts with defensive emotions, in order to prevent his/her physical body from feeling, thereby exaggerating emotional needs. This type of individual is also very prone to sublimation of the sex drive.

**EMOTIONAL SUGGESTIBILITY** – A suggestible behavior characterized by a high degree of responsiveness to inferred suggestions affecting the emotions, and a restriction of physical body responses; usually associated with hypnoidal depth.

**EMOTIONAL SEXUALS** – Feel their sexual responses inwardly. They use their emotions to draw attention away from their bodies. Their priorities in life are career, hobbies, relationships and family, then a mistress and friendships.

**PHYSICAL SEXUALS** – Project their sexual responses outwardly. They use their bodies to draw attention away from their emotions, which they feel are vulnerable. Their priorities in life are their relationship, children, friends and hobbies, then career.

**ENVIRONMENTAL HYPNOSIS** – A state of hypersuggestibility triggered when an individual is in the presence of an overabundance of message units coming from their environment. This causes the person to try to escape the intense input. A kind of "walking hypnosis."

**EXPECTATION** – The state of mind in which the individual expects something to happen. Expectation triggers imagination and greatly facilitates the hypnotic induction, especially with Emotionally suggestible subjects.

**EXTRAVERBAL COMMUNICATION** – Communication by physical gestures or movements that infer a suggestion to an individual, according to his interpretation. Body language is an example.

**EYE ACCESSING CUES** – An NLP technique of observing the unconscious eye movement to determine if a subject is mentally seeing images, hearing sounds, engaging in self-dialogue or experiencing kenisethic feelings.

**EYE FASCINATION INDUCTION** – This is used when a Hypnotherapist notices during the interview that a client's eyes tend to fade or blink repeatedly. The client is asked to stare at an object above eye level. The therapist speaks rapidly and paternally, telling the client their eyelids are getting heavier and beginning to close. When they close, the therapist touches the client on the forehead, says "deep sleep", then pushes the client's hands off his lap to create a loose, limp feeling in his body.

**FEAR OF FALLING AND LOUD NOISES** – According to the Kappasinian Theory of Mind (T.O.M.), babies are born with only two fears, that of loud noises and of falling. All other fears are learned.

**FIGHT OR FLIGHT REACTION** – A primitive and involuntary reaction that is triggered during danger or anxiety, in order to protect oneself or to escape from danger.

**FRAME** – NLP construct implying a way of perceiving something or to set a context (As if Frame, Context Frame, Outcome Frame, Rapport Frame, Backtrack Frame).

**GLOVE ANESTHESIA** – A type of hypnoanesthesia where the client's hand is made to feel numb, and they are told that numbness can be transferred to any part of their body that feels discomfort.

**HALLUCINATION** – A sensory experience arising apart from any corresponding external stimulation; a mental image taken for a reality.

**HOMEOSTASIS** – A state of equilibrium. What the body returns to when the parasympathetic nervous system is activated to respond to the fight/flight mechanism of the sympathetic nervous system.

**HYPERSUGGESTIBILITY** – A state of waking hypnosis and exaggerated suggestibility to influencing factors in the environment, especially to negatives; possibly the greatest cause of all emotional and physical problems.

**HYPNODRAMA** – The process of acting out a role in the hypnotic state, which can be used for increasing talents or reducing the effects of earlier traumas in the client's life.

**HYPNOIDAL** – A light stage of hypnosis, usually associated with

Emotional suggestibility; also used to refer to the state of consciousness which is passed through in the transition from sleep to waking, and vice versa.

**HYPNOSIS** – An altered state of consciousness which results in an increased receptiveness and response to suggestion. While associated with relaxation, hypnosis is actually an escape from an overload of message units, resulting in relaxation. Hypnosis can be triggered naturally from environmental stimuli as well as purposefully from an operator, often referred to as a hypnotist.

**HYPNOTHERAPIST** – A therapist who utilizes hypnosis as a primary tool for assisting clients to achieve their goals. A Hypnotherapist often differs from others therapists by focusing on the role of subconscious behaviors and influences on the client's life.

**DEFINITION OF HYPNOTHERAPIST** – 079.157-010 – In 1973, Dr. John Kappas, Founder of HMI, wrote and defined the profession of a Hypnotherapist in the Federal Dictionary of Occupational Titles...

*"Induces hypnotic state in client to increase motivation or alter behavior patterns: Consults with client to determine nature of problem. Prepares client to enter hypnotic state by explaining how hypnosis works and what client will experience. Tests subject to determine degree of Emotional and Physical suggestibility. Induces hypnotic state in client, using individualized methods and techniques of hypnosis based on interpretation of test results and analysis of client's problem. May train client in self-hypnosis conditioning."*

**HYPNOTIST** – A person skilled in the technique of inducing the hypnotic state in others. Hypnotists are often associated with the use of hypnosis for entertainment.

**IDEOMOTOR RESPONSE** – A response emanating from an individual's subconscious mind via the central nervous system. Such a response is a way of avoiding judgments of the conscious mind. Examples: handwriting, index finger raise while in hypnosis.

**IMAGERY/HYPNODRAMA** – Imagery is a feeling and experiential state. Unlike visualization, which relies only on the idea of "seeing" something in the mind's eye, imagery uses all five of the senses. Hypnodrama, like Psychodrama, allows a client to act out subconscious conflicts in a safe environment in an attempt to vent and resolve them. However, in Hypnodrama the client does this internally, so there may be less possible embarrassment. Also, since Hypnodrama uses imagery, there is more access to the emotions and the senses than typical Psychodrama. The more senses that are tapped, the better able to re-experience the conflict.

**INCONGRUENT BEHAVIOR** – When a person's sexual behavior is the opposite of his suggestible behavior, or when his outward expression is inconsistent with his actions.

**INDUCTION** – The technique of hypnotizing a person. The patter used can be either maternal or paternal; either one sends message units to the brain, preparing the subject to enter the hypnotic state.

**INFERRED SUGGESTION** – A suggestion given that contains a message other than the immediately obvious one. Usually, the underlying meaning is not immediately understood consciously by the subject, but he will have a delayed reaction to it. It is especially effective with Emotionally suggestible subjects.

**INHIBITORY PROCESSES** – The processes that allow a person to deal with himself and with his external environment in a rational and civilized way. When inhibitory processes are disorganized, heterohypnosis results; when they are organized, self-hypnosis takes place.

**INTELLECTUAL SUGGESTIBILITY** – The type of suggestibility in which a subject fears being controlled by the operator and is constantly trying to analyze, reject, or rationalize everything the operator says. With this type of subject, the operator must give logical explanations for every suggestion and must allow the subject to feel that he is doing the hypnotizing himself.

**KNOWNS (PAIN/PLEASURE PRINCIPLE)** – Knowns represent pleasure, in that they are things we have associated or identified before. A Known may be either positive or negative but is accepted by the Subconscious because it has been experienced before. Conversely, Unknowns represent pain, or physical or psychological threats that have not been associated or identified before.

## LAWS OF SUGGESTIBILITY

**Reverse Action** – The most common law, it's sometimes referred to as Reverse Psychology. A person will respond to the stronger part of a suggestion if the alternative presented is considerably weaker.

**Repetition** – It is represented by the fact that the more we do something, the better we become at it. By repeating suggestions in hypnosis, the stronger the suggestive idea becomes.

**Dominance** – The use of authority or that of being an authority figure to "command" the client to accept a suggestion. Capitalizing on one's position as "therapist" or by using an authoritative tone are two approaches to apply the Law of Dominance.

**Delayed Action** – When a suggestion is inferred, the individual will react to it whenever a jogging condition or situation that has been used in the original suggestive idea presents itself.

**Association** – Whenever we repeatedly respond to a particular stimulus in the presence of another, we will soon begin to associate one with the other. Whenever either stimulus is present, the other is recalled. The post suggestion to re-hypnosis works under this law.

**LIFE SCRIPT** – Formed from the positive and negative associations we've made throughout our life and stored in our subconscious mind. This is reflected in a person's present life situation.

## LITERAL/INFERRED SUGGESTIONS

**Literal Suggestions** – A direct suggestion with no underlying meaning; used primarily with Physically suggestible subjects.

**Inferred Suggestions** – A suggestion given that contains a message other than the immediately obvious one. Usually the underlying meaning is not immediately understood by the client consciously, but he/she will have a delayed reaction to it. It is especially effective with emotionally suggestible clients.

**MAGIC 30 MINUTES –** The last half-hour before sleep, when a person's mind is overloaded and is in a natural state of hypnosis. Something taken into the mind at this time goes into the precognitive stage of dreaming, instead of the venting stage.

**MATERNALISM –** A soft, gentle, lulling, rhythmic approach to hypnosis. A progressive relaxation uses the maternal approach.

**MENTAL BANK –** A tool used to reinforce many types of therapies and speed the progress in such areas as; procrastination, motivation, goal attainment, prosperity, weight loss, smoking, etc. It is a powerful means of affecting the subconscious mind using the synergistic approach of belief, daily reinforcement, scripting, time of day, and dreams.

**MESSAGE UNITS –** All of the input sent to the brain by the environment, the physical body, and the conscious and subconscious minds. When too many message units are received (as in a life threatening emergency), a state of anxiety results.

**MISDIRECTION –** Appearing to be guiding someone into one area, with the intention of directing him into another. It can be used effectively as a deepening technique in hypnosis.

**MODALITIES –** A hypnotic modality is anything that attempts to control or modify human behavior through the influence or creation of belief systems.

**NEURO PATHWAYS –** Every time we think a thought, make a movement, experience something, this is transformed into electro-chemical energy which is then stored in the brain. We create pathways that allow the energy to travel in a similar fashion each time it is triggered. The more it is triggered, the easier it is for the energy to go that route. This is how habits and behavior, both good and bad, are created.

**NEUTRALIZING SUGGESTION –** A suggestion that is made to counter the effect of previous suggestions that have been given to a subject. Neutralization is especially important in stage work.

**ORGASM –** A resolution to the sex act, which is accompanied by contractions, bodily warmth, spasmodic shivering, genital moisture, and a feeling of release. Orgasm is distinguished from climax, which is a less dramatic, though still potentially pleasurable, resolution of the sex act. The terms used in this way are generally applied only to women, with orgasm usually characteristic of the Physically sexual female and the climax of the Emotionally sexual female.

**PARATAXIC DISTORTION –** This occurs when we respond to a person or situation in a distorted way. We are not responding to the situation or person, but rather to what they subconsciously trigger in us.

**PARIS WINDOW –** Used to widen the perspective of the client, so that he or she can see their problem from more than their own viewpoint. The window is a four-paned one, where three panes contain a question for the client. The questions are, 1). How do you feel about the problem? 2). How do you think others feel about your problem? 3). How do you feel about how others feel about your problem? 4). This pane contains the answer to the client's particular problem based on their newfound perspective.

**PATERNALISM –** The authoritarian approach to inductions and therapy, using a rapid patter with commanding, or even demanding, words.

**PATTER –** A rhythmic series of words in a semi-monotone or monotone, spoken either slowly or rapidly, causing stimulation of different senses and leading to the hypnotic state.

**PERSUASIVE SUGGESTION –** A suggestive idea that gives the subject a logical reason to respond. Persuasive suggestions are particularly effective with Intellectually suggestible subjects.

**PHYSICAL SEXUALITY –** A type of sexual behavior in which the individual reacts to physical stimulation as a defense to protect his/her emotional behavior, thereby exaggerating the need for physical acceptance and gratification.

**PHYSICAL SUGGESTIBILITY** – A suggestible behavior, characterized by a high degree of responsiveness to suggestions affecting the body and a restriction of emotional responses; usually associated with cataleptic stages or deeper.

**POST HYPNOTIC SUGGESTION** – An example would be the command of "deep sleep."

**POST SUGGESTION TO REACTION** – A suggestion given, to be carried out after the subject has awakened from the hypnotic state.

**POST SUGGESTION TO REHYPNOSIS** – A suggestion given for re-hypnosis, to take place when a certain stimulus is seen, heard, or felt by the subject; creates a rapid response to re-hypnosis.

**POWER WORDS** – The dominant words projected from the operator to the subject that impart some type of direction or control. (Example: "Deep sleep!")

**PRE-INDUCTION** – An introduction to hypnosis to prepare the subject for the induction. It should include an explanation of hypnosis and an idea of what the subject can expect to experience in the state. It addresses any fears and misconceptions the client may have, all the while building up message units.

**PRIMITIVE MIND** – A human being's primitive brain, with which a person will react whenever threatened beyond the point where he/she can reason. This primitive brain produces the fight or flight response, the unthinking impulses of self defense, or any other rapid reactions without reason.

**RAPPORT** – The operator/subject relationship, in which the subject has faith and confidence in the operator, and the operator has concern for the client.

**REACTIONAL HYPNOSIS** – Repeatedly awakening the subject and re-hypnotizing him with a post-suggestion to re-hypnosis. An effective method of achieving depth in hypnosis.

**RESISTANCE** – A sign that a person is running into his/her limiting programming and having an affect on it.

**REVERSAL** – A suggestion given with a very weak challenge and a strong negation, as in challenging the eyelids: Your eyelids are closed. You may try to open them, but the more you try, the more difficult it becomes.

**SECONDARY GAIN** – A reason, primarily subconscious, why a person continues to perform a certain behavior.

## SELF-HYPNOSIS – HETERO HYPNOSIS

**Self-Hypnosis** – A hypnotic state that is self-created.

**Hetero-Hypnosis** – A hypnotic state that is created by another person, including the listening to of tapes or CDs.

**SHOCK INDUCTION** – A very rapid conversion into hypnosis. Shock inductions are primarily used only in emergencies or possibly to "jar" a client when in therapy.

**SOMNAMBULISM** – The deepest stage of hypnosis, where the subject responds with amnesia, anesthesia, negative and positive hallucinations, and complete control of the senses. This type of subject usually has 50% Emotional suggestibility and 50% Physical suggestibility.

**STAGES OF AMNESIA** – There are 3 stages of Amnesia (found at the Somnambulism Depth)

**First Stage** – The individual will exhibit between 20% to 40% spontaneous amnesia.

**Second Stage** – The individual will exhibit approximately 60% spontaneous amnesia.

**Third Stage** – The individual will respond to all types of suggestions. This person will exhibit 80% or more spontaneous amnesia, remembering almost nothing that occurred while in hypnosis.

**STAGES OF LOSS** – There are five stages a person must go through to completely deal with a loss. Not every individual will display all the symptoms nor in the same time or manner. The stages are 1). Denial, 2). Anger, 3). Bargaining, 4). Grief, 5). Resolution.

**STOP MECHANISM** – A technique used in hypnosis to call attention to a behavior or thought a client may do or have in the future. When this thought or behavior arises they will hear in their mind "NO!" The Hypnotherapist reinforces this suggestion by stating the thought or behavior the client may have, snapping their fingers and saying "NO!" to the client. This is reinforced several times with the client repeating it to themselves silently but strongly. An example would be if the client thought about lighting up a cigarette when they were trying to or had already quit.

**SUBCONSCIOUS** – The 88% of our mind that is mostly below the level of our awareness. The part of our mind responsible for reflexive action, ideomotor responses, and contains the positive and negative associations we've made throughout our life.

## SUGGESTIBILITY (EMOTIONAL/PHYSICAL/INTELLECTUAL)

**Emotional Suggestibility** – A suggestible behavior characterized by a high degree of responsiveness to inferred suggestions affecting emotions and restriction of physical body responses; usually associated with hypnoidal depth. Thus, the Emotional person learns more by inference than by direct, literal suggestions.

**Physical Suggestibility** – A suggestible behavior characterized by a high degree of responsiveness to literal suggestions affecting the body, and restriction of emotional responses; usually associated with cataleptic stages or deeper.

**Intellectual Suggestibility** – The type of hypnotic suggestibility in which a subject fears being controlled by the operator and is constantly trying to analyze, reject, or rationalize everything the operator says. With this type of subject the operator must give logical explanations for every suggestion and must allow the subject to feel that he is doing the hypnotizing himself.

**SYMPATHETIC – PARASYMPATHETIC** – The two divisions of the Autonomic Nervous System.

**Sympathetic** – When activated causes physiological changes to occur, preparing the body for fight/flight.

**Parasympathetic** – A self-regulating, stabilizing system that brings a person back to a state of balance, or homeostasis.

**SYSTEMATIC DESENSITIZATION** – The process of inducing a relaxed state in the client and then having him/her visualize or imagine an event that was traumatic to him or her in the past. The relaxation then becomes the dominant force, and as the client begins to relate to being relaxed and calm while relating to the trauma area, he/she allows for removal or desensitization of the trauma.

**THEORY OF MIND** – The mind is divided into four areas; all of which must be affected to enter the state of hypnosis. The four areas are;

**The Primitive Area** – Part of the subconscious and established from birth. It contains the fight/flight response and the fears of falling and loud noises.

**The Modern Memory Area** – Also a part of the subconscious and contains all of a person's memories (Knowns).

**The Conscious Area** – Formed around the age of 8 or 9, and is the logical, reasoning, decision making part of the mind.

**The Critical Area** – Also formed around the age of 8 or 9, filters message units and accepts or rejects them from entering into the Modern Memory. If the Critical Area is overwhelmed, it breaks down, activating fight/flight, causing a hypersuggestible state, that is, hypnosis.

**VENTING DREAMS** – The third stage of dreaming (after Wishful Thinking and Precognitive Stages), characterized by the mind's attempt to vent, or release, the overload of message units accumulated during the day.

*This page intentionally left blank.*

# INDEX

*This page intentionally left blank.*

# HMI BOOKSTORE

The HMI Bookstore provides streaming video, audio, MP3 downloads, DVDs, CDs, books and eBooks about hypnosis, hypnotism, hypnotherapy, self-hypnosis, behavioral reprogramming and self-improvement programs.

For a complete HMI Bookstore Catalog visit https://Hypnosis.edu/Bookstore or call Panorama Publishing toll free in the U.S. at **800-634-5620**. From outside the U.S. call **001-818-758-2751**.

---

## Success is not an Accident: The Mental Bank Concept

John G. Kappas, Ph.D. – $24.95 – eBook $19.95
https://Hypnosis.edu/Books/Mental-Bank-Concept

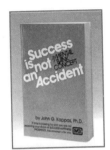

The Mental Bank program, developed by Dr. John Kappas and the staff of the Hypnosis Motivation Institute (HMI), represents the culmination of 45 years experience in the field of subconscious and behavioral reprogramming.

The text "Success is not an Accident" explains in easy-to-follow steps the five synergistic elements of the Mental Bank Program and how to get them working in your life in less than five minutes per day.

The Mental Bank Program is a dramatic demonstration of how your subconscious mind is a goal machine, driven to achieve whatever it is programmed for.

The Mental Bank Program puts you in the driver's seat for programming your subconscious mind to achieve SUCCESS, HAPPINESS and PROSPERITY, easily and effortlessly.

---

## The Mental Bank Ledger

John G. Kappas, Ph.D. – $14.95
https://Hypnosis.edu/Books/Mental-Bank-Ledger

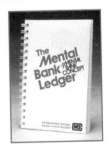

The Mental Bank Ledger is the workbook that accompanies the self-improvement program outlined in the text "Success is not an Accident: The Mental Bank Concept."

The Mental Bank Ledger also accompanies the Mental Bank Video/DVD instruction course as well as the live presentation of the Mental Bank Program.

The Mental Bank Ledger is easy to use and a must for the effortless application of the Mental Bank Program.

For those utilizing the powerful Mental Bank Program, the Mental Bank Ledger is their nightly companion and partner is success.

**Note:** Prices are subject to change without notice. Please visit the online HMI Bookstore for the latest products and prices. https://Hypnosis.edu/Bookstore/

# HMI BOOKSTORE

## Relationship Strategies

John G. Kappas, Ph.D. – $24.95 – eBook $19.95
https://Hypnosis.edu/Books/Relationship-Strategies

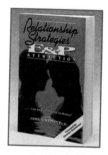

Having a successful relationship is the most important and yet for many the most difficult aspect of our lives. Why some people struggle more than others and why some people are more successful than others in relationships is perhaps the most important question that the behavioral sciences can strive to answer.

For more than 30 years the Hypnosis Motivation Institute, under the direction of Dr. John Kappas, has been examining the question of how much of our relationship patterns are dictated by our subconscious mind? How much of our behavior in relationships has been programmed from childhood. What role does the subconscious mind play in who we choose in relationships and why?

Dr. John Kappas' Relationship Strategies: The E&P Factor reveals simply and clearly how the subconscious mind dictates who we choose for partners in our relationships and why we repeat many of the same patterns over and over again. Learning to recognize these subconscious traits in ourselves and in our partners begins a three step process of understanding, predicting and finally shaping behavior so that the powerful forces of the subconscious mind can begin working for us instead of against us in building successful relationships.

## Professional Hypnotism Manual

John G. Kappas, Ph.D. – $27.95 – eBook $19.95
https://Hypnosis.edu/Books/Hypnotism-Manual

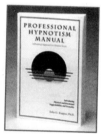

Dr. John Kappas' Professional Hypnotism Manual is more than just another book about hypnosis. It is instead a comprehensive system for looking at people's behavior as a whole under an umbrella that is best described as "subconscious behaviorism."

In this book, Dr. John Kappas completely redefines our understanding of hypnosis and how it works with his "Message Unit Theory of Hypnosis", as well as introduces his revolutionary model of "Emotional and Physical Suggestibility and Sexuality."

The "E&P" model provides hypnotherapists with a road map of how each client requires a unique delivery of hypnotic suggestions and a novel understanding of the wide range of subconscious behaviors and responses between individual subjects.

These new concepts, along with the countless gems of practical wisdom contained in this book, have earned the book distinction as a classic text in the hypnosis of modern history.

**Note:** Prices are subject to change without notice. Please visit the online HMI Bookstore for the latest products and prices. https://Hypnosis.edu/Bookstore/

# HMI BOOKSTORE

## Kappas Book Package 1
Complete Kappas Book Package – $89.95 – Savings of $28.75
https://Hypnosis.edu/Bookstore/Packages/#PUBPKG001

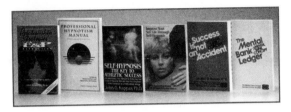

- PUB001 – Professional Hypnotism Manual (eBook Included)
- PUB002 – Relationship Strategies (eBook Included)
- PUB003 – The Mental Bank Concept (eBook Included)
- PUB004 – The Mental Bank Ledger
- PUB005 – Improve Your Sex Life with Self-Hypnosis
- PUB006 – Self-Hypnosis: The Key to Athletic Success

## Kappas Book Package 2
Kappas Book Package – $71.95 – Savings of $18.80
https://Hypnosis.edu/Bookstore/Packages/#PUBPKG002

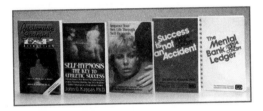

- PUB002 – Relationship Strategies (eBook Included)
- PUB003 – The Mental Bank Concept (eBook Included)
- PUB004 – The Mental Bank Ledger
- PUB005 – Improve Your Sex Life with Self-Hypnosis
- PUB006 – Self-Hypnosis: The Key to Athletic Success

**Note:** Prices are subject to change without notice. Please visit the online HMI Bookstore for the latest products and prices. https://Hypnosis.edu/Bookstore/

# HMI BOOKSTORE

## Kappas Book Package 3

Complete Mental Bank Package – $39.95 – Savings of $29.90
https://Hypnosis.edu/Bookstore/Packages/#PUBPKG003

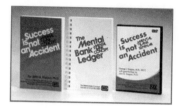

- PUB003 – The Mental Bank Concept (eBook Included)
- PUB004 – The Mental Bank Ledger
- VSI001 – The Mental Bank Seminar

---

## Kappas Book Package 4

Mental Bank Book and Ledger Package – $29.95 – Savings of $9.95
https://Hypnosis.edu/Bookstore/Packages/#PUBPKG004

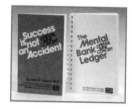

- PUB003 – The Mental Bank Concept (eBook Included)
- PUB004 – The Mental Bank Ledger

---

## Kappas Book Package 5

Double Mental Bank Ledger Package – $21.95 – Savings of $7.95
https://Hypnosis.edu/Bookstore/Packages/#PUBPKG005

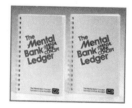

- PUB004 – The Mental Bank Ledger

# HMI BOOKSTORE

## Improve Your Sex Life
## Through Self-Hypnosis

John G. Kappas, Ph.D. – $12.95 – eBook $8.95
https://Hypnosis.edu/Books/Improve-Sex-Life

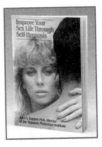

**Improve Your Sex Life Through Self-Hypnosis** spells out, in clear, simple language, self-hypnosis techniques that have been tested by the author in thousands of private therapy cases.

Within these pages, Dr. John Kappas shows you how to focus your thoughts and forget everything but the pleasure of the moment.

He takes a fresh new look at: How crippling past experiences can cause current problems. How you can end (or avoid) such common sexual problems as premature ejaculation, impotence, lack of lubrication, and tightening of the vaginal muscles through self-hypnosis.

Complete with special questionnaire that measure your sexuality and suggestibility, Improve Your Sex Life Through Self-Hypnosis offers a practical, effective way for anyone to experience the full joy of sex. Read it today!

---

## Self-Hypnosis:
## The Key to Athletic Success

John G. Kappas, Ph.D. – $12.95 – eBook $8.95
https://Hypnosis.edu/Books/Self-Hypnosis

Now you can improve your athletic skills whether you are a beginner, a skilled amateur, or a professional. Here's a book to help you be the best athlete you can be – through self-hypnosis!

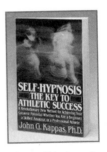

**Self-Hypnosis: The Key to Athletic Success** teaches you the self-hypnosis techniques that will help you develop the same confidence and motivation that enable professional athletes to achieve their peak performances.

The author, a practicing hypnotherapist who has helped thousands of top athletes, reveals that simple will power is not enough; you must learn to get in touch with the inner resources that determine your motivation and performance. In these pages, you'll learn to do just that – with a clear, easy-to-follow program that works for any and all sports!

If you're a professional athlete striving to achieve your fullest potential, or just a weekend golfer or jogger interested in improving your score or your mileage, this book will get you in touch with a source of strength and excellence you never knew you had!

**Note:** Prices are subject to change without notice. Please visit the online HMI Bookstore for the latest products and prices. https://Hypnosis.edu/Bookstore/

# HMI BOOKSTORE

## Facing Today and the Future Through Self-Hypnosis

John G. Kappas, Ph.D. – CD $14.95 – MP3 $9.95
https://Hypnosis.edu/Audio/

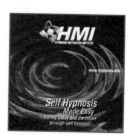

Dr. John G. Kappas, has devoted his professional life to furthering the understanding of the uses of hypnosis.

In addition to being the founder of America's First Nationally Accredited College of Hypnotherapy, he is also the founder and first president of the Hypnotherapists Union Local 472 AFL-CIO and the American Hypnosis Association (AHA).

"Facing today and the future through self-hypnosis" spells out, in clear, simple language, self-hypnosis techniques that have been tested by the author in thousands of private therapy cases.

Introducing Dr. Kappas' model of Emotional and Physical Suggestibility, you will learn your own personalized formula to maximize your potential with self-hypnosis. Practice with an easy-to-follow conditioning exercise and guided hypnotic induction.

---

## Free Hypnosis Training Videos and Online Self-Improvement Classes

- **HMI Web TV – Hypnotherapy Television 24/7**
  https://Hypnosis.edu/WebTV/

- **Success is not an Accident: The Mental Bank Program**
  https://Hypnosis.edu/Streaming/Mental-Bank/

- **Relationship Strategies: The E&P Attraction**
  https://Hypnosis.edu/Streaming/EP/

- **Hypnosis in History**
  https://HypnosisInHistory.com/

---

## HYPNOSIS MOTIVATION INSTITUTE

18607 Ventura Boulevard, Suite 310
Tarzana, California 91356-4158 USA
HMI Bookstore: 800-634-5620 • Outside U.S. 001-818-758-2751
In-Person Training: 800-479-9464 • 818-758-2747
Online Training: 800-600-0464
Website: https://Hypnosis.edu/

**Note:** Prices are subject to change without notice. Please visit the online HMI Bookstore for the latest products and prices. https://Hypnosis.edu/Bookstore/